Workouts for Seniors Over 60

9-Minute Full-Body Guided Exercise Routines to Vastly Improve Flexibility, Strength, Balance, and Relieve Joint Pain

Robert Balazs

Table of Contents

A Free Gift to all My Readers!

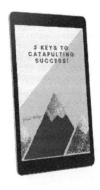 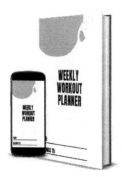

As a thank you and to help you on your fitness journey, I would love to send you a free copy of my **weekly planner** so that you can plan your workouts, as well as my eBook titled *5 Keys To Catapulting Success*!

To receive your complimentary copies now, please visit www.robertbalazs.com.

Introduction

Experiencing low energy and limited mobility can be a thorn in the flesh, especially when you have your grandchildren around. It's the desire and pleasure of every grandparent to make their grandkids' stay with them as enjoyable as it can be and you are not an exception. The pain that comes with hearing them say, "Granny, can you please play this game with us?" while you know you are not fit enough to do so is unbearable.

Pain in the joints, knees, and back can also make life quite difficult if you are a senior, not to mention potential health issues that creep up on you over time. As you go through this book, you will discover the important role that is played by exercise, should you decide to incorporate it as part of your everyday lifestyle and you will understand how working out can benefit you in a positive way. The fully illustrated, step-by-step exercises provided in this book are hand picked to target all of the vital muscles in your body leaving you jovial, energetic and healthier in the long run.

This book is a great handbook for seniors of all experience levels and is for those wanting to experience the magic behind a full-body workout. If you want to get some new moves, or are looking for a structured program to get you started this book will do just that. If you are new to working out, you will not go wrong with this book as it is designed to be low impact and scalable. With consistency and determination, you will learn to love the way it makes you feel. Get ready to explore and be one of the fittest seniors around, with improved flexibility, balance, strength, and less joint pain!

Meet the Author

Robert Balazs was born in Canada and moved to Scandinavia by the age of 19. Robert has always had a passion for exercise and sports, in addition to helping other people. Over the years Robert has assisted hundreds of clients, the majority of which have positive feedback with regards to how exercise has impacted their lives. Robert is also a certified personal trainer with over a decade of experience within training. Due to his passion for helping others achieve their goals, Robert says, "There is no better thing than seeing people's struggles start to get better over time." Robert Balazs saw the need to write this book because he observed that only a few senior citizens actually have a structured training program in their daily routine. Worse still, even fewer senior people know the countless benefits that are associated with a workout-conscious lifestyle. One of the main reasons why Robert wrote this book is because he is so keen to reach as many senior citizens as possible, with the ultimate aim of contributing to their improved everyday life.

Chapter 1:

Learning About Your Body

As you age, your body undergoes certain processes that you have no direct control over. These biological events are a natural part of the aging process in human beings. In this chapter, we will focus on enlightening you about what happens in your body as you age. This knowledge is crucial because it enhances your understanding with regard to why training should be a crucial part of your everyday lifestyle. The information that you will get in this chapter will give you reasons that serve as a footing for engaging in an active lifestyle. Simply put, after reading this chapter, you will see how much you have been missing out by living a life that is not centered around being active. However, the better part of the story is that it's never too late to start making it right and give your body the proper care that it deserves. Remember, "Knowledge is power."

Aging and the Muscles, Bones, and Joints

As human beings age, there are changes that happen to their posture and walking patterns. Usually, these changes are attributed to alterations that take place in the bones, joints, and muscles as years go by. We are going to delve deeper into some of such changes in this chapter.

Aging and Your Bones

The skeleton that supports your body is made up of bones that are connected together through joints. When you are young, your bones are strong and so is the skeleton. As a result, your body posture is straight and uncompromised. This state changes as your body tends to get weaker with age. You might find it progressively difficult to keep your spinal cord straight. In fact, you may experience immense pain in your back if you try to. In some cases, the bones don't only get weaker as you age, they might become brittle, and this can result in them potentially being easier to break. While bones can sometimes break as a result of injuries, brittle bones simply fracture without any reasonable cause. This, of course, significantly affects your walking patterns and posture.

The bones that make up your spinal cord are known as the vertebrae. These bones are arranged in such a way that there is a gel-like substance called hyaluronic acid located between each of them. The role of this substance is to cushion the vertebrae, as well as maintain the size of your trunk. The trunk is the region of your body that is located below your head and just before your legs. As ages catch up with you, the gel-like cushion loses fluid, thereby making the vertebrae appear shorter. The result of this change is a shorter trunk. The mineral content of the spine bones also reduces with age. All these changes contribute to a curved and compressed spinal cord, something which is quite common among the elderly.

Conditions Associated With the Bones

Now that you have an idea of some of the things that happen in your body as you age, let's have a quick rundown of the conditions that tend to emerge as you age. In this section, we will focus more on the conditions that affect your bones.

- **Osteoporosis:** It is normal for bone mass and density to reduce with a corresponding increase in age. This is especially true for women who are in their menopause. Science has it that bone density tends to remain stable for age ranges between 25 and 50 years (Johns Hopkins Medicine, 2022). Beyond 50 years of age, bone formation begins to take place at a pace that is slower than the rate at which they break down. This results in reduced mass and density of the bones in the long run.
- **Osteophytes:** Osteophytes happens when finger joints lose their cartilage and the bones get slightly thicker.

Aging and Your Joints

Walking patterns are also affected by unhealthy joints. Your flexibility and ease of movement is a factor of good and able joints. The reason why your bones do not rub against each other as you walk is the presence of synovial membranes and fluids that surround the joints. These fluids lubricate the joint area to reduce any form of friction that might possibly occur. The amount of synovial fluid that is available in your joint areas may reduce as you grow older. This means that the probability of your bones brushing against each other as you move becomes elevated. Walking becomes more difficult and even painful. This is part of what takes away the joy of most senior citizens as they fail to move without external support.

Your joints are also cushioned by what is known as cartilage, which covers the ends of your bones. They are there to further protect your bones from rubbing against each other. The older you grow, the more these cartilages begin to wear away, thereby exposing the ends of your bones. This condition is called arthritis and it adds to the uncomfortable feelings that senior citizens might experience in their joints as they walk. Loss of cartilage is quite common on the hip and knee joints. In joints around the shoulders, minerals may accumulate on the joints, a process that is known as calcification.

Aging and Your Muscles

Your muscles also play major roles in enhancing your movements. They provide the strength and force that you need for movement to happen. However, aging comes with reduced vigor as the muscles grow weaker, too. Medically, the condition in which muscle function is lost as a result of aging is called 'sarcopenia'. This word originates from the Greek language where *'sarcos'* refers to flesh and *'penia'* means loss (Physiopedia, 2019). Sarcopenia is characterized by loss of muscle energy, accompanied by the eventual reduction in muscle functionalities.

People with sarcopenia have reduced numbers of satellite cells. These cells are highly involved in the regeneration and repair of muscle cells, both of which lead to muscle growth (Physiopedia, 2019). This partly explains why the loss of lean body mass occurs as you age.

Coordination of muscle movement takes place in the brain. The changes that your muscles and joints undergo as you age affect your brain's ability to coordinate movements. As a result, you will feel weak and your speed of movement is impeded. Let's discuss more on the changes that take place in the muscles as humans age.

Reduced Muscle Mass

Aging is usually characterized by atrophy. This is a scenario where muscle tissue is lost, leading to reduced lean body mass, which subsequently reduces function. Worse still, losing about 40% of lean mass has fatal consequences in your body. It is thought that genes might have something to do with the changes that take place in the muscles as people age (MedlinePlus, 2017). They determine the rate at which this process happens. Muscle changes tend to take place earlier in men than it does in women.

In older individuals, especially those above 50 years old, the lost muscle tissue is replaced by increased fat mass. These structures are, unfortunately, non-contractile. This decrease in muscle mass, alongside the accumulation of fat tissue reduces flexibility and impedes your movement. Please note this change in muscle mass was observed in the lower limbs of adults through a scientific research study (Henwood, 2008).

Another change that is worth mentioning is the deposition of an age-related pigment that is known as lipofuscin, in the muscle tissue. This pigment brings about a variety of changes, including the shrinking of muscle fibers and the slower replacement of muscle tissue. In cases where the muscle tissue is replaced, this happens with tough fibrous tissue. This causes body parts to appear bony and thin, especially the hands. The muscles become less able to contract, so they are less toned.

Lower Muscle Strength

Your muscles are powered by what is known as muscle fibers. These fibers power your movements and other activities that you might engage in. Even your day-to-day activities and chores are made possible by the existence of these fibers in your muscles. Now, as you continue to age, these fibers are reduced significantly and because of this, your muscle strength is also reduced. This explains why it becomes increasingly difficult for you to complete some tasks as you grow older. The same things that you once used to carry in your hands without any struggle might feel heavy for you as you age.

According to one study, changes that are related to strength reduction usually affect mobility, walking ability, upper extremity function, speed, as well as sit-to-stand and balance performance (Kahraman et al., 2019). The results that were presented from this study showed that significant changes in muscle fibers take place within one-year periods, in senior citizens.

Changes in muscle fibers occur in two major forms. These are

- **Changes in the size of the actual fibers:** Some muscle fibers reduce in their cross-sectional size as well as in their numbers. These changes negatively impact muscle strength as highlighted earlier.
- **Changes in size and number of motor units:** The proper functioning of the muscle fibers is enhanced by the presence of motor neurons. These are nerve cells that coordinate the functioning of the muscle fibers. In all human beings, loss of nerve supply and its restoration take place constantly. These two processes are referred to as denervation and reinnervation, respectively. In the elderly, denervation happens at a rate that is faster than that of reinnervation, thereby causing poor function of the muscle fibers.

Exercise: One of Your Best Solutions

The discrepancies in functionality and ability that come with aging can be quite frustrating at times. However, the good news is that these are not without a solution. A study that was published in PubMed revealed that people who engage in strength training exercises do away with frailty, weakness, and other conditions that come as a result of aging (Seguin and Nelson, 2003). The research in this study shows that strength exercises revamp muscle mass and strength, in addition to preserving your bone mass and density, too. Balance will be enhanced, thereby reducing the chances of falls and avoidable injuries. Please note that according to the study, you should work out at least two or three times a week for you to enjoy the aforementioned benefits of strength training.

The research by Rebecca and Mirriam Nelson also showed that strength training can combat some of the common diseases that are associated with aging. For instance, they reported that the risk of suffering from osteoporosis and other chronic conditions like type 2 diabetes, heart disease, and arthritis is also significantly reduced. Not only that, you will sleep better when consistently working out. Some psychological issues like depression and related stress are kept at bay when you sleep better.

Another study that was published in the Medicine and Science in Sports and Exercise Journal revealed that there is a reduction in the age-accelerating effects of inflammation due to strength training (Csatari, 2021). Researchers divided a total of 103 previously sedentary people into three groups. Some of them went into aerobic training, others into strength training, and the last group was the control. A reduction in the blood levels of an inflammation marker referred to as C-reactive protein was seen in both exercise groups. For the resistance training group, numbers reduced 32%, double as compared to the aerobic group. The reduction in the inflammation marker for both training groups, therefore, shows that the incorporation of these workouts will produce remarkable results when it comes to the health of seniors.

Simply put, exercise is one of the easiest ways through which you can prevent, slow down, or manage problems that are linked to bones, muscles, and joints. It helps you to regain flexibility, strength, and balance. The results from the aforementioned study led to the conclusion that strength training can be prescribed to senior citizens as a tool for dealing with some of the inconveniences that are caused by old age. In response to such a call, this book will provide you with training ideas that work, while making sure that is safe, too.

We recommend that you book an appointment with your family or personal health professional before you start your training. This is meant to further enhance your safety. As you do your strength training, we also encourage that you eat a well-balanced diet that is rich in calcium sources. For those who are above the age of 70, consuming about 1200 milligrams of calcium daily is a great idea (Physiopedia, 2019).

It's Never Too Late to Start!

There is no proper time to commence training—any time is tea time! If you haven't yet started experiencing the aging symptoms that we described in this chapter, you can start now to reduce their impact on your body. You can be that grandpa or grandma who is still capable of doing things on their own, even at old age. If some of the aging symptoms have already caught up with you, again, it's all good. There is no need to get discouraged and wish you had come across this book at an earlier stage. First, you still have what it takes to reduce further unpleasant symptoms. Second, some issues can be rectified. For instance, you can still regain your strength and energy. Some aches like the back pain will cease to be as severe as they might have been before. Exercising is for life so it doesn't matter when you decide to start. You can begin now!

Chapter 2:

Getting Started

The purpose of this chapter is to get you prepared for starting your exercises. We will look at all the things that you need for a successful and effective workout program. Not only will we discuss the material preparations that you need, but we will also highlight the mental orientation that creates a winning mindset. Remember, winning starts in your mind, before it manifests in the physical. By the time you get to the end of this chapter, you should have gathered all you need to get the ball rolling.

Type of Clothing

Not all clothing is very supportive of all postures when you train. This is why you need to know the right types of clothing for you. This helps to get the best out of your workouts. In this section, we will discuss what you should wear when you exercise.

Athletic Shoes

Athletic shoes are a necessity if you are serious about taking on training sessions. When you get these, you will realize that they are worth the money that you would spend on them. We recommend that you choose shoes with a flat sole as they will provide a stable base. Obviously, you would want shoes that are comfortable and that do not make you feel itchy after each session. Select shoes that are flexible for your forward, backward, and sideway strides. Your shoes should offer some form of support as you assume different postures. They should also have a cushioning effect that protects the skin on your feet.

As is the case with clothes, the type of shoes that you choose might depend on the form of workouts that you would want to do. Of course, the other general features that we mentioned before will apply to all types, no matter the type of exercise that you would like to engage in. However, take note of these differences. If your workouts will involve running, light shoes that are both flexible and supportive are what you need. A thinner sole would be a better option, as it is more likely to make the shoe lighter. If you are going for strength training, get sneakers that are rubber-soled and relatively light.

Be sure to replace your shoes constantly if need be or when the need arises. If the sole is worn out, get a new shoe to keep up with the requirements that make your training as enjoyable and beneficial as it should be. Finally, here is another important consideration that can easily be forgotten—get the right shoe size! Getting the wrong size can be the worst mistake that can make you dread training time so get that right before anything else.

Breathable Clothes

You will certainly need clothes that will not make you feel too hot, which is the reason why we recommend breathable clothes. You are more likely to sweat when you work out. For this reason, the clothes that you wear should have the ability to draw sweat from your body and also dry out quickly. Clothes that are made of synthetic fabrics are more likely to have this characteristic, especially those made of polypropylene and polyester. Wool clothes can also be a good option

(MedlinePlus, 2022). To make it easier for you, check for clothes that are tagged as "moisture-wicking."

You also need quick-drying fabrics for your socks. This will assist in avoiding blisters due to the accumulation of heat. To be on the safe side, go for socks that are made using the polyester blend, among other special materials.

Cotton absorbs sweat but it dries out at a relatively slow rate. The latter makes cotton unsuitable for clothes that you use when you exercise. Due to the fact that cotton stays wet when it absorbs sweat, it can make you feel cold when you work out in colder seasons.

The fit of your clothes is as important as the material that is used to make them. Your clothes should fit you in such a way that they should not hinder your moves when you exercise. Your clothes should fit you in such a way that they should not hinder your movement when you exercise. Simply put, your clothes must not be too tight or baggy. You should feel comfortable in them. Clothes that are too big for you can catch on exercise equipment. This can derail your focus, thereby negatively affecting the training session, overall

In most cases, the fit of your clothes may depend on the type of exercise that you intend to do. For instance, you might need slightly loose clothing when you intend to walk or engage in gentle yoga and strength training. Form-fitting clothes that are a bit stretchy are a great option for swimming, biking, running, and advanced yoga moves. Wearing combinations of tight-fitting and loose clothes is also a possible option. Here is a good example: you can wear a tight-fitting bottom or shorts, alongside a loose-fitting T-shirt. Whatever is comfortable for you will work, just make sure it absorbs sweat and dries quickly.

Other Resources

In addition to proper clothing for your training session, there are other things that you should keep handy. Remember, we need to make your sessions the best that they can be. Find out more resources that are of paramount importance as far as your workout sessions are concerned.

Water Bottle

Training will have you sweating out. The water that you lose as you exercise needs to be replaced regularly. This is why you need a water bottle with you as you go through each session. Presumably, you already know that drinking water is an important component of keeping your body healthy. It is even more important when you work out. Besides replacing the sweated out water, hydrating yourself by drinking water as you workout will maintain your energy levels exactly where you want them to be.

Jay Cardiello, a trainer at Gold's Gym Fitness Institute once said, "Just look at the parallels between oil in a car and water in a body — a car can't run without oil, a body can't run without water" (Tucker, 2019). Before, during, and after your training, you should be constantly sipping your water to keep yourself hydrated and in "tip top shape."

Just a general tip — aim to drink half of your body weight each day and that should also determine the size of the bottle that you should buy (Tucker, 2019). In essence, drink at least 65 ounces of water if you weigh 130 pounds.

Mat or Blanket

For beginners, one of the questions that would pop into their minds when we talk about exercises is, "How do I know the mat that is best for me?" Well, this is the question that we are going to answer now. Generally, any type of mat or a regular blanket should work. However, if you want something that is more customized, you can buy mats that match the type of exercises that you intend to do. Another important factor when you choose a mat is the size. Just make sure your mat can support you and you can fit on it. Considering size and purpose, shorter mats are more appropriate for stretching after doing your workouts. You can also use these mats for abs exercises. If you want to do longer yoga and fitness sessions, longer mats are a better option.

You might also need to consider the thickness of your mat. Generally, thicker mats are more comfortable. Moreover, they are less likely to get damaged. If you are able to get a mat that is about 0.7 centimeters thick, you are good to go. The make of the mat is also crucial. Make sure the surface of your mat is plain and a bit slippery. Such a surface is easier to clean. The underside of your mat should be preferably non-slip, with a gripping effect on the floor. You wouldn't want a mat that would be moving out of position as you do your exercises.

Dumbbells

Dumbbells will give a special touch to your workouts, and help you scale your workouts if they are too easy for you.f you don't have dumbbells in your home, that's no big deal because you can still use water bottles Yes, they do work, too!

Considerations to Make When Buying

Please note that dumbbells are created differently. Let's have a quick look at some of the considerations that you should make when you purchase the dumbbells that you can use for your home workouts.

Fixed Versus Adjustable Weights

As the name suggests, fixed weights cannot be removed or adjusted, so you have to be sure about the weight that you need before you purchase them. If you need different weights, then you have to buy multiple pairs and this generally takes up a lot of space. Therefore, when you opt for fixed weights, make sure you have enough storage space as well. Fixed weights are more appropriate to beginners as far as lifting weights is concerned. For most of the exercises that we will describe in this book, the fixed weight will work well for you.

Adjustable dumbbells have functionality that allows you to alter the weight. They have a dial system that you can use to set the amount of weight to what you want. These weights also have a safety lock to make sure that the weights do not slip and fall on you. Adjustable dumbbells are the best option if you do not have enough storage space. Buying them also saves money, considering that you won't have to purchase different sets separately. Adjustable weights are more suitable if you lift bigger weights so they are usually used by seasoned weight trainers.

The Shape of the Dumbbells

The shape of the dumbbells matters too. You will normally find these in two shapes, which are, a circle and a hexagon. Choosing the shape that is more appropriate for you depends on what you want to use them for. Circle dumbbells can easily roll on the floor so if you are going to do exercises where you use them as a platform, they are not your best choice. Rather go for hexagon-shaped ones in that case. Circle dumbbells are preferable when you are using them as an ab roller, for example.

Material of the Dumbbell

Usually, dumbbells are made of metal, rubber, and urethane. If you are working out at home, rubber and urethane ones are better because they are less likely to damage the floors.

Chair

If some of the exercises you are performing are too difficult, you might need a chair for support. For simpler exercises, seniors that find it difficult to stand even for a few minutes, a chair would also come in handy. The same applies to exercise routines that are a bit longer. You can start off without a chair and then use it later. Any chair that you have in your home will do, preferably the ones without armrests and a solid sitting surface.

Towel

Keep your towel close as you will need to wipe off some sweat during your exercises. Sweat can be irritating if you don't wipe it off. If you are working out with others, you don't want them to see you dripping sweat everywhere. Besides, sweat accumulating on your body produces an unpleasant odor.

Prepare Your Body

Having gathered all the other things that you need as we have described in this chapter, you also need to prepare your body for the workout. One of the most important things that you should keep in mind is how you fuel and refuel your body before and after the workout session, respectively. For a well-planned workout session, you should know what and when to eat before you exercise and when you are done.

Just like a car would need gas before it takes off, your body also needs proper food to fuel it. Starting your workout on an empty stomach is not a good idea, yet you should not eat immediately before the workout either. Your pre workout meal should be consumed between one and three hours prior to your workout. As a rule of thumb, the closer you get to your workout, the more you need to avoid eating. You certainly don't want to experience stomach issues when you are in action.

When you eat, aim for a meal that is balanced in nutrients. Your meal should include carbohydrates and lean protein. Don't eat much fiber and fats as these are digested at a much slower rate. Therefore, they might upset your stomach during your workout. Low-fat Greek yogurt with berries, alongside a small salad that is topped with chicken, is a great pre-workout meal. You can also eat a Turkey-and-Swiss cheese sandwich, together with low-fat chocolate milk. Feel free to explore other options out there that match your preferences!

There is no rush. Focus on proper form and controlling your breathing. You got this!

Wear a 'Winning' Mindset

For your workout endeavors to produce desired results, you need to develop a winning mindset. Such a mindset will keep you going even when the going gets tough. A winning mindset will keep you focused on your goals whatever they may be. A winning mindset is the equivalence of a growth mindset, which is quite the opposite of a fixed mindset. Individuals who have a growth mindset are good, available, and willing learners. They believe that apart from the set of abilities that you were born with, you can still learn other things and improve yourself. When you develop a growth mindset, challenges stop hindering you from your dreams. Instead, you will learn to see opportunities in challenges and let it fuel you. Instead, you will learn to see opportunities in challenges and work so hard to improve.

Contrary to the growth mindset is the fixed one. Those with fixed mindsets believe that abilities are limited to the set of talents that one is born with. With this kind of mindset, there is little to no hope for improvement. Individuals with fixed mindsets are prone to giving up. If challenges come their way, they retreat or quit. You wouldn't want such a mindset if you want this book to work for you in the way that is intended.

Starting to exercise is not going to be necessarily easy, but very manageable. You will, therefore, need a growth or winning mindset to get the desired results. Some exercises may not be as comfortable, especially as you start but that should not stop you. Think about what exercising will do for your body, children, grandkids, and all the people around you. You can and you will!

So, how can you develop and nurture a winning mindset? Here are some pointers that will work for you if you put them into practice:

- **Focus on getting better at it:** Your third day exercising will never be the same as the first day. There are a lot of other things that you will master as you go. Therefore, do not let today's failures halt you. Always aim to improve.
- **Winners are not your focus, winning is:** This is one of the things that you should keep in mind. People who lose spend much of their time focusing on what other people are doing, as well as comparing themselves with the people around them. That's the wrong focus. Remain fixed on winning. We are all different but do the best that we can to get to the winning mark. Focus on becoming stronger and more flexible than before, if that is your goal. If you want to do away with or manage joint pain, your focus should be glued on attaining that.
- **Cultivate patience:** Whatever it is that you intend to get out of your exercise routines, it will require some time for it to manifest. For instance, joint pain will not disappear in your first workout session. You will start to notice positive changes and feel better as time progresses. For this reason, you will definitely need a lot of patience for you to see expected results.

How Does It Work?

This is a nine-minute workout that is designed for seniors, especially seniors. This workout will target every major muscle group in the body. It will also incorporate light stretching, balance, and cardiovascular training. Stretching and warm-up are not included in the nine minutes. Before every workout, stretching and warm-up exercises should be performed to better prepare the body for the actual main exercises that are a part of this workout.

This set of workouts is designed to be scalable either up or down so that it can be performed at any fitness level. Each exercise is to be performed for 40 seconds, followed by a 20-second rest. Keep going until you have gone through all eight exercises. For each muscle group, there are multiple options that are presented. This means that you can switch from one exercise to the other to keep things interesting. Always consult a physician before performing workouts as a measure to ensure that your health is safe. The workouts that are described in this book are designed such that you can do them on a daily basis. I encourage beginners to start with three days a week with a goal of gradually working their way up doing the exercises every day.

Stretching

Prior to the workout session, it is highly recommended to do the stretches in this book to warm up your body. Stretching comes in two main forms, which are dynamic and static stretching. In this book, more emphasis is put on dynamic stretching because static stretching can hinder your performance. You will understand why this is so as you continue to read through this section.

Static Stretching

Static stretching involves stretching your muscles to the furthest point that they allow you and then maintaining the position for some time. This type of stretching has its own benefits but it is not good for pre-workout warm-ups. Here are some of the benefits of static stretching:

- It is effective in improving your flexibility and the range of movement for your joints.
- It keeps tears and serious muscle strains at bay.

So you can see from these benefits that static stretching is not completely bad. There are instances when it is more appropriate, just not before the exercises that we will describe in this book. This is because prolonged static stretching can switch your muscles off and this negatively affects your overall performance during exercises. One scientific study reported that each time a stretch is held for more than 60 seconds, the potential to produce muscle force is reduced by approximately 4.6% (Behm et al., 2016). It is better to do a static stretch for a few seconds, say 45 seconds, and then to dynamic stretches soon afterward. This way, you increase flexibility without losing the touch of high performance during workouts.

Dynamic Stretching

Dynamic stretching describes the type of movements where you move a joint in an active manner, past its round of movement, and without having to hold the stretch. Each dynamic stretch can be repeated about 12 times. Arm circles are a good example of a dynamic stretch. This stretching method improves the way your muscles function so they will be more active when you then have to do the actual set of exercises that you intend to do after warming up. According to research, dynamic stretching is an awesome tool when it comes to muscle strength, flexibility, and even the overall performance when you are jumping or sprinting (Ellerton, 2018).

Let's look at more insights about the benefits of dynamic stretching:

- **Enhancing muscle performance:** When you do dynamic stretching, your agility, speed, and acceleration are improved. Overall, this leads to the betterment of your activity during workouts.

- **Improved flexibility:** The muscles that are around your joints need to be stronger. This, along with an increased range of motion, enhances your flexibility.
- **Better body awareness:** Dynamic stretching tends to mimic the movements that you will do during your planned set of exercises. This makes this type of stretching an effective full-body workout. Your muscles become better prepared for the exercises, well before you actually start.

The World's Greatest Stretch

Now, as an example of a dynamic stretch, we will describe how you can do the world's greatest stretch. In this exercise, we are trying to gain a greater range of motion, limber up, and pump blood into the muscles that we are going to train. Please perform five repetitions of each variation and do the same on the opposite side. To do the world's greatest stretch, follow these steps and enjoy:

1. Stand, with your feet placed slightly apart.
2. Now, move the left foot slightly ahead of the position that it was in when you were standing.
3. Go down until the knee of your right leg touches the floor, while the left one simply bends accordingly without moving the foot.

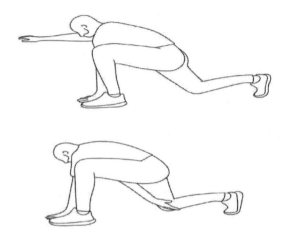

4. Stretch both hands and let them touch the ground. They should be at the right side of the left leg, side-by-side with it.
5. Stretch your right hand toward the front as if you are reaching for something and then bring it back so that it touches the inner side of the right knee while everything else remains in the same position.

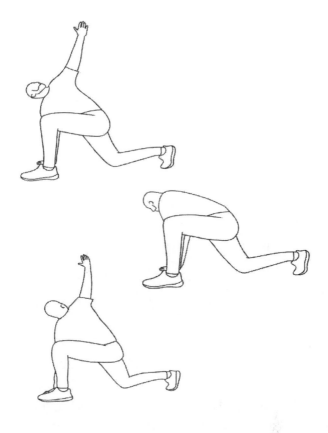

6. Now, lift the right hand up high toward the ceiling, while the left one remains on the floor. As you put the right hand back to the floor, raise the left one in the same way.

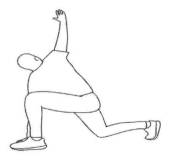

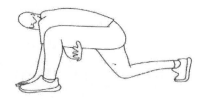

7. Still, in the same position, stretch the right hand toward the ceiling again and allow it to pass through between your two legs as it stretches toward the left.
8. After completing all three stretches on one side, switch to the opposite leg and perform the same thing on this side.

Chapter 3:

Active Warm-Up

You might have been told time and time again that you have to warm up your body before working out. However, do you know the positive effects of pre-workout warm-ups? If not, there is no need to worry. This chapter will enlighten you on the reasons why warming up is a crucial part of preparing for your workout. You will also get tips and tricks as well as exercise recommendations that you can incorporate in your warm-up sessions. Get more serious with warming up after reading this chapter.

Why Warm-Up?

When you are warming up, you are simply doing exercises at a pace that is a little slower than you would for the actual exercises. The intensity of the exercises is also lower. One of the most important reasons why warm-ups should be part and parcel of your exercise routines is that they prepare your body for heavier, more rapid, and more demanding exercises. You don't want to shock your body by suddenly taking it from rest to raid and vigorous exercise. Instead, you should take it step by step.

Warming up is a way of steadily revving up your circulatory system. The temperature of your body gradually rises, while blood flows to the muscles at a much faster rate. This means that your heart will begin to beat faster and your breathing rate increases, too. A higher breathing rate increases the transportation of oxygen to your muscles while taking away the carbon dioxide from respiratory processes. When this happens, your muscles will contract much more easily, thereby making it easier for the exercises to serve their purposes. By the time you start to do the actual exercises, body processes would have been optimized to match the body's higher demands during more vigorous workouts. The heart, for example, won't be strained by a sudden change into rigorous activity.

Pre-workout warm-ups can also reduce muscle soreness. This in turn helps to reduce the risk of injury during your workouts. The elasticity of your muscles improves when you warm up. This also contributes to reducing the possibility of straining a muscle as you exercise.

As mentioned earlier, the mind plays a crucial role in the whole workout process. Warm-ups are another way to prepare your mind for the exercises that you want to do. With a well-prepared mind, you are better motivated to achieve your goals for working out. No matter how difficult some movements might seem to be, the likelihood of giving up is very slim when you are mentally prepared for the exercises. Therefore, as you do your warm-ups, keep reminding yourself of the fact that your body needs the exercise. Also, think about what you stand to gain from exercise. Be determined to succeed!

Have you ever paid attention to how stiff and rigid your body can be after a period of rest? It is quite difficult to engage in exercises right away as your muscles aren't flexible enough. The pre-workout stretches enhance the flexibility of your muscles both on a short- and long-term basis. The increased movement of the blood toward the muscles makes them relax more so they can better endure the workouts that you intend to do.

Let's Go Practical!

The warm-up session in this book includes three exercises. All the exercises should be performed before the commencement of every workout. Each warm-up exercise should be performed for 40 seconds, followed by a 20-second rest period. Please note that each warm-up exercise has to be performed one time to fully complete the warm-up. This means that in total the warm-up will be 3 minutes long. We are, therefore, going to describe how to perform these warm-ups in this section.

Marches

The goal of this movement is to raise your knees as high as possible, without going past the range that makes you feel comfortable as you do it. With this exercise, you are warming up your hip flexors and engaging your ankles because of the balance aspect. This warm-up exercise also engages your core, in addition to getting your heart pumping at a faster rate. If it's not possible for you to perform the exercise while standing, you can do it by sitting on a chair and lifting your knees.

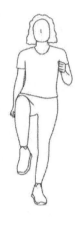

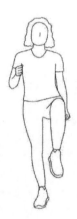

To perform the 'marches,' follow this procedure:

1. Stand in an upright position with your feet slightly apart, just like you would when you are about to walk. Make sure your arms are at your sides.

2. While the left foot remains on the floor, lift your right knee up toward the ceiling as much as you can. Also, lift your left arm by bending it at the elbow at the same time. When you move your arm, it should assume the position it takes when you are running.

3. As you bring back the right foot to the floor, simultaneously lower your left arm as well, so that you reassume the position in (1).
4. Repeat steps (2) and (3) but this time you lift the left knee and the right arm.
5. Keep alternating between the left and right knee accordingly for 40 seconds.

Air Boxing

When air-boxing, the muscles that are activated are your shoulders, core, and arms. It is possible to scale down to sitting on a chair and boxing if it's not possible to perform the exercise while standing. The targeted body parts will still be activated, whether you are standing or seated.

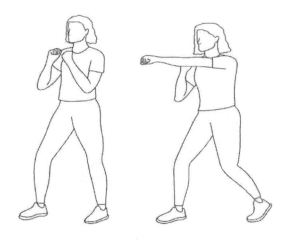

Air boxing is quite easy to perform as you will see from these steps:

1. First, stand with your feet slightly apart, before moving your left foot forward. Raise both arms as if you are about to fight and make sure your palms are fisted. Look straight ahead as if you are looking at an opponent. You can call this position the "boxing stance."

2. Hit the air, at shoulder height, with the right fist, while you withhold the left one. Repeat this action as you

alternate hands. Be sure to keep your feet in place as you do so.

3. Repeat the procedure as many times as possible, within the 40-second range.

Step Back and Reach

This is another exciting warm-up. The purpose of this exercise is to enable you to gain mobility in your back and core, as well as enhance your balance. We can't skip the fact that this set of warm-up movements will pump blood to your whole body and get you ready. If for any reason this exercise is too difficult to be performed standing, you can perform it while sitting. All you have to do is sit on a chair and raise your hands over your head and stretch as far as possible.

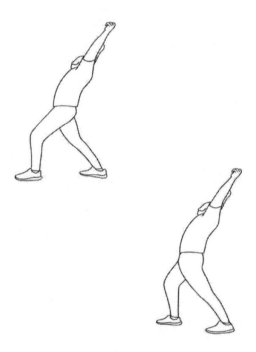

This procedure shows you how to do the "step back and reach" warm-up exercise:

1. Stand in an upright manner, making sure that your hands are at your sides.
2. Stretch your right leg behind your body as much as is comfortable for you and place this foot firmly on the floor.
3. Raise both hands up high toward the ceiling and simultaneously stretch them backwards.
4. Bring back the right foot to its starting position, right beside the left foot.
5. Now, stretch the left leg, just as you did for the right one in step 2 above.

6. Repeat step 3 before bringing back the left foot to its original position.
7. Keep alternating between the right and left legs until your 40-second timer rings.

Chapter 4:

Legs and Lower Back

Most seniors tend to have problems with their legs and lower back, especially as they grow older. This chapter will help you to understand the muscles that are affected as years go by. Not only that, you will be enlightened on the reasons why regularly exercising our posterior chain is of paramount importance. To help you start to incorporate the habit of working out your lower back and legs, we will describe the step-by-step practical exercises that you can do on your own.

Lower Body Muscles

Muscles work hand-in-hand with your bones to ensure that the body has the support that it needs. The roles of muscles in your body fall into two major categories. First, there are muscles that are primarily involved in body movement. These are the muscles that aid and control your flexibility. Second, other muscles aid body positioning and support. These are the muscles that are responsible for keeping your posture.

In this section, we will discuss the different muscles that make up the lower body, together with their functions. As you read on, you will notice that the position where the muscle is located determines its functions. This means that knowing where a muscle stretches to and from is an easy and quick way of determining whether it is involved in movement or support. With this knowledge and understanding, you can then exercise with an enlightened and purposeful mind. Don't worry much about some of the big names that you will hear in this section; what these words are referring to is what matters most.

As you explore the muscles in your lower body, please note that muscles that stretch across two joints are prone to becoming stiff, especially when you lead a sedentary lifestyle. If these muscles become stiff, the flexibility of the affected joints is negatively affected and this might reduce the efficient functioning of the joint area overall.

Leg Muscles: The Overview

Legs are a major part of the lower body muscles. Leg muscles can either be upper or lower muscles, based on their location on your legs. The ones that are found in the region of the leg that stretches from your waist down to your knees are the upper leg muscles. Again, your guess is as good as mine—lower leg muscles stretch from the knee going downward. The front region of both the upper and lower leg area is described as the anterior, while the back part is called the posterior. All the muscles on your legs work together in helping you to jump, walk, run, and even tip-toe. These muscles collaborate with your bones, ligaments, and tendons in accomplishing all the tasks that we mentioned.

Upper Leg Muscles

Your upper leg is made up of two main groups of muscles. These are the quadriceps and hamstrings. There are four muscles that constitute the quadriceps. Just a point to note—quadricep muscles are among the largest and strongest of all the muscles that are in your body. The main role of quadricep muscles is in straightening your leg. Here are the four muscles that are part of your quadriceps:

- **Vastus medialis:** This muscle is located on the inner side of your thigh. It appears like a teardrop in shape. The vastus medialis stretches along your thigh bone up to your knee.
- **Vastus lateralis:** This muscle is found on the outer side of your thigh. Being the largest muscle among the quadricep muscles, the vastus lateralis stretches along the thigh bone, until it reaches the kneecap.
- **Vastus interdius:** This is the deepest muscle among all the muscles of the quadriceps. The vastus interdius is located in such a way that it is between the Vastus lateralis and vastus medialis muscles.
- **Rectus femoris:** This is the muscle that makes it possible for you to raise your knee. The rectus femoris also aids the flexibility of your hips and thighs. This crucial muscle is attached along your hip bone.

The hamstrings are found at the back of your thighs. When you bend your knees, your hamstrings are at work as they are well-positioned for this purpose. There are three main muscles that are worth mentioning when you talk about your hamstrings. All of these muscles stretch from just below your buttocks to your shinbone. Please note that these three hamstring muscles are located behind the hipbone. Let's discuss these muscles (Roland, 2020):

- **Semimembranosus:** This muscle starts from your pelvis, going down until it reaches your shinbone. This is the muscle that enables you to rotate your shinbone, extend your thigh, as well as flex your knees.
- **Biceps femoris:** This spans the region between your lower hip bone and your shinbone. The bicep femoris enables you to extend your hip, in addition to flexing your knee.
- **Semitendinosus:** This muscle is positioned between the Biceps femoris and Semimembranosus. Its main roles are in helping you to rotate the shinbone and

thigh with enhanced ease. This muscle also contributes to assisting you to extend your hip.

Lower Leg Muscles

The region between your knee and ankle is what we are referring to as the lower leg. The calf, which is behind the shinbone, contains the main muscles of the lower leg. Let's delve into the details of these main lower leg muscles in this section.

- **Soleus:** Running down your calf, is a muscle called the soleus. This muscle is the reason why you are able to lift your foot from the ground when you are walking. The soleus also helps you to maintain a stable posture when you are standing.
- **Gastrocnemius:** The gastrocnemius muscle is large, as it stretches from your knee, right to the ankle. With the help of this muscle, extending your knee, foot, and ankles is possible and easier, too.
- **Plantaris:** The plantaris muscle is small and is found at the back of your knee. There are some people, about 10% of the world's human population, who do not have this muscle (Rolaand, 2020). These people do not experience any sort of lack or loss as the contribution of the plantaris in flexing the knee is very minimal.

Lower Back Muscles

Your lower back is part of the lower body and it is mainly responsible for supporting your upper body. As you might be already aware, you have a spinal cord on your back. This structure supports your whole body, as you assume different postures. The proper function of your spine is enhanced by the presence of back muscles. There are basically three types of back muscles that play crucial supportive roles to the spine. These are:

- **Extensor muscles:** You will find these muscles attached to the back of your spinal cord. A good example of an extensor muscle is the erector spinae, which is located on the lower back. The role of this muscle is to keep the spine in position by holding it up. Generally, extensor muscles play a vital role in helping you to stand and carry objects, whether heavy or light.
- **Flexor muscles:** Unlike the extensor muscles, the flexor ones are attached to the front of your spinal cord. Flexors are the structures behind your ability to bend forward, flex your back, as well as lift objects.
- **Oblique muscles:** Attached to the sides of your spine, you have the oblique muscles. The presence of these muscles enables you to rotate your spine. Oblique muscles also help you to maintain your posture.

The Posterior Chain

The structures at the back of the spine and legs make up what is known as the posterior chain. We have already discussed some of the muscles that are located in these regions, including the calf, hamstring, and erector spinae muscles. Posterior chain muscles play a major role in enhancing your strength and speed, even as you go about your everyday business.

The muscles that are part of the posterior chain make movement remarkably easier. In some instances, the movement would be completely impossible if these muscles were absent. Now, let's look at it this way. Imagine a scenario where the posterior chain muscles are present but are unable to perform their function as expected—sometimes, it's as good as if they are not there at all. Movement either becomes reduced, painful, or impossible. This is what happens when you disregard exercising your posterior chain muscles, especially as you grow older. Your muscles will grow rigid.

Working out strengthens the muscles of the posterior chain. It reduces the probability of sustaining injuries. Moreover, when you exercise these muscles, you increase the chances of enjoying the benefits that are associated with their presence. Your spine, knees, and hips become more stable, which is less likely to happen in senior citizens who do not exercise. The best part is that you don't have to look any further for workouts that strengthen your posterior chain. They are provided in the next section.

Workouts for the Lower Body

In this section, you will get step-by-step instructions for different exercises that are great for your lower back and legs. Please note that you should choose two leg exercises that you can perform during each nine-minute workout session.

Air Squats

This exercise is mainly training the front of your thighs, that is, the quadriceps. If balance is an issue in this exercise, place a chair in front of you and hold the chair as you squat down. For an easier variant, you can grab a chair, sit down, and stand up while still focusing on holding the same form. If the exercise is too easy for you, consider holding dumbbells to make the exercise heavier.

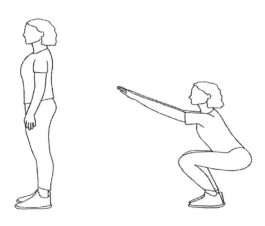

To perform the air squats, follow the steps that are outlined below:

1. Stand in place, making sure that your feet are about shoulder-width apart. Flare feet slightly out.
2. Stretch your hands straight out in front of you, so that they are perpendicular to the rest of your body. This helps you to attain and keep balance as you carry out your exercises.
3. Squat down, while making sure that your feet are planted on the floor. Your knees should move in the same direction as your feet as you go down. Press through your heels and squat down as low as you can. The ultimate goal is to go down to a 90-degree angle,

but if this is too difficult just go down as far as is possible for you.
4. Once you get to the squat level that you can maintain, push yourself up so that you assume the starting position again.
5. Repeat the procedure for the full 40 seconds.

Good Mornings

This exercise is mainly targeted at training the back of your thighs, that is, the hamstrings, glutes, and lower back. If you feel that the exercise is too difficult for you, you can perform it while sitting on a chair.

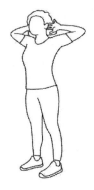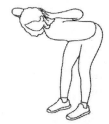

Here are the steps that you can follow to do this exercise:

1. Stand in place so that your feet are about hip-width apart from each other. Your toes should be pointing forward. Slightly bend your knees and be sure to maintain this throughout the exercise.
2. Knot your hands together and place them behind your head.
3. Start the movement by pressing your hips back, while bending forward to bring your upper body and chest down towards the floor. You should go far enough for you to feel a slight stretch in the back of your thighs.

4. Come back up to the start position by bringing your upper body up again.
5. Repeat and enjoy!

Standing Side Leg Raise

The purpose of this exercise is mainly focused on training the side of your glutes and thighs. It is totally understandable if the exercise feels too difficult for you. Don't stop though—just do it while supporting yourself by placing your hands against the wall.

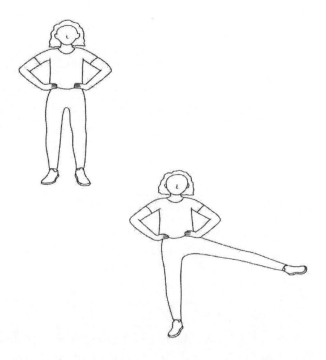

To do this exercise, follow this procedure:

1. Assume your normal standing position, making sure that your hands are holding your waist. Your feet should be facing forward. Again, be sure to keep your legs straight throughout the exercise.
2. Lift one leg directly out to the side as far as you can, while squeezing your glute.
3. Bring the lifted leg back down and immediately lift the other one toward the other side.
4. Keep alternating your legs as described in steps 1 and 2 above.

Lying Hip Thrusts

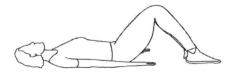

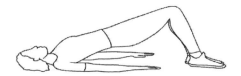

This exercise is meant to train your glutes, hamstrings, and lower back. You can perform it by following this procedure:

1. Place a mat or blanket on the space where you are going to perform your workouts. Lay down on your mat or blanket, with your back on the floor. Your hands should lie at your side, with the palms face down on the floor.
2. Push your feet up towards your upper body. Do this until your knees form a 90-degree angle against your upper body.
3. Thrust your hips straight up in the air, while your shoulders and head remain stuck to the floor. When you lift your hip area, your body, from your shoulders to the knees, should form a straight line that appears slanted. Squeeze your glutes on the way up and lower back down again to the ground.
4. Repeat the procedure.

Lunges

This is one of the exercises that can significantly improve your stability and mobility. The lunges work out your hips, legs, as well as your back by targeting the larger muscles in these parts.

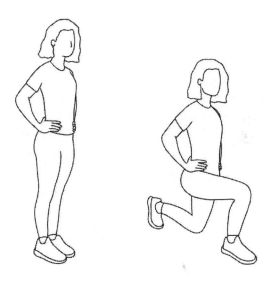

Follow this procedure to do the lunges:

1. Assume a standing pose and place your hands on your waist.
2. Step in front with your left side foot.

3. Lower your right knee down until it touches the floor and raise yourself up again.
4. Return the left foot to its initial position and immediately step forward with the right foot.
5. Repeat step 3 but this time lowering the left side knee.
6. Repeat.

Superman

This workout is a good complimentary exercise for leg raises and sit-ups that mainly focus on strengthening the abdominal muscles that are located at the front of your body. This is because 'superman' primarily impacts the lower back muscles. Your glutes and hamstrings will also benefit from this workout.

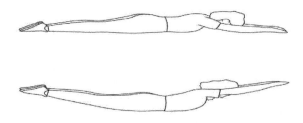

The steps for performing this exercise are outlined below:

1. Lie down on your belly with your toes touching the floor. Hold your hands together while they remain on the floor, while your head is off the ground.
2. Simultaneously lift your "held together" hands, together with your shoulder area and lower legs.
3. Bring the lifted parts back to the floor again and repeat step 2.

Chapter 5:

The Back

The back plays a fundamental role in maintaining your posture. There are many activities that are highly dependent on the strength of the muscles that are found in the back. Although it holds such importance, the back muscle is among the ones that are greatly affected by aging. Working out the back muscles can greatly reduce the rate at which these natural processes take place. The focus of this chapter is on enlightening you on the muscles that are found in the back. More importantly, this chapter is packed with exercises that target back muscles. With such a combination of knowledge and practice, you will exercise with 'understanding.'

Muscles of the Back

The muscles that are found in the back are classified into three groups, which are, superficial, intermediate, and deep muscles. The superficial ones are those muscles that are highly involved in shoulder movements. The intermediate back muscles participate in enhancing thoracic cage movements. The back muscles that have a role to play in vertebral column movements are referred to as deep muscles. The vertebral column is the axis that is central in all skeletons of vertebrates. The deep muscles are also called the intrinsic muscles because their development starts in the back. This is contrary to the development of intermediate and superficial back muscles, whose development does not originate from the back. For this reason, these two muscles are known as extrinsic back muscles.

Superficial Back Muscles

Superficial back muscles stretch from the vertebral column to the bones that are found in your shoulder. These shoulder bones are the scapula, clavicle, and humerus. By virtue of them being attached to the bones of the shoulders, superficial back muscles are highly involved in enhancing upper limb movements. In this section, we will discuss more on the different muscles that fall under the superficial back muscle category. These include the trapezius, levator scapulae, and latissimus dorsi.

- **Trapezius:** This muscle is flat and broad, assuming a triangular shape. The trapezius is unique for being the most superficial among all the muscles that are found in the back. The trapezius's upper fibers are responsible for raising the scapula, in addition to rotating this shoulder bone when the arm is abducted. The retraction of the scapula is aided by the middle fibers of the trapezius. The lower fibers exert a slight pull on the scapula.
- **Latissimus dorsi:** The latissimus dorsi covers a remarkably large area of the lower back, which is where its origins are. This muscle is the reason why you are able to extend and adduct your upper limb. The latissimus dorsi is also responsible for promoting rotation of the upper limb.
- **Rhomboids:** The rhomboid muscles exist in two forms, which are, the major and minor. The rhomboid major is also attached to the scapula, a position that enables it to play its roles in retracting and rotating the scapula. Attached at a similar position as the rhomboids, the medial border of the scapula, the

rhomboid minor is also involved in retracting and rotating the scapula.

- **Levator scapulae:** This muscle appears like a strap. It originates from the neck and stretches down to the scapula, where it is attached. The main purpose of the levator scapulae is to elevate the scapula.

Intermediate Back Muscles

Only two muscles make up the intermediate group of muscles. These are the serratus posterior superior and serratus posterior inferior. Both muscles play vital roles in elevating and depressing your ribs. This function is enhanced by their strategic positioning as they are attached to the rib cage while originating from the vertebral column. It is also believed that the intermediate back muscles contribute to respiratory functions (TeachMeAnatomy, 2022).

- **Serratus posterior superior:** This muscle is thin and it assumes a rectangular shape. Its location is deep under the rhomboid muscles that are on the upper back. The serratus posterior superior is the one that elevates ribs two to five.
- **Seratus posterior inferior:** The serratus posterior inferior is stronger and broader, compared to the serratus posterior superior. It is found beneath the latissimus dorsi. This muscle is responsible for depressing ribs nine to twelve.

Superficial Muscles

Also known as the spinotransversales, superficial muscles play crucial roles in aiding neck and head movement. Two muscles, which are, the splenius capitis and splenius cervicis, are the members of the superficial muscles category. These muscles are in the neck where they spread over the deeper neck muscles. The splenius capitis rotates the head to the same side and so does the splenius cervicis.

The Positive Effects of Training Your Upper Back

Even to younger people, consistently maintaining a good posture can be a challenge. The intensity of this problem tends to increase as one grows older. Poor postures are usually apparent when people are sitting in schools, workplaces, or other gatherings. After all has been said and done, the good news is that exercise can significantly improve your posture. Think of how many times you might have tried to consciously maintain an upright posture yet you keep forgetting once in a while and find yourself in that hunched position. It's quite difficult. The approach of training your back helps you to build up strength in your back and shoulder muscles. This way, the back muscles are strong enough to keep you in an upright position. Simply put, when the muscles in your shoulders and back are strong, keeping them up requires less effort on your side.

Apart from assisting you to maintain a good posture, a stronger back is a plus when you are running around and completing everyday tasks. All tasks involving some level of pulling and pushing, will not give you much of a hard time when your back muscles are strong. Some things like lifting groceries out of the car into your house naturally become more difficult as you age, but regularly training your back muscles will help combat this. Other simple, unavoidable tasks like opening and closing doors can appear demanding when you have weak back muscles.

Workouts for Back Muscles

As far as your starter pack for exercises that target the back muscles is concerned, look no further. This section presents a set of exercises that help you feel renewed and strong each time you engage in them. Please note that for the purpose of the nine-minute workout, choose two back exercises from this section each time you do your workout session.

Reach and Pull

When you do this exercise, you should feel its impact on your upper back and shoulders. It is a good exercise for helping you to maintain a good posture. It is possible to perform this exercise while seated on a chair.

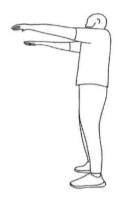

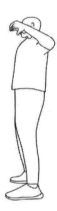

Please, find the step-by-step outline on how to do this exercise here:

1. Assume the starting position by standing with your feet at shoulder width. and a slight bend in your knees.

2. Raise your arms to shoulder height and stretch them toward the front of your body. This will appear as if you are reaching for something.

3. Row your arms back to neck level while keeping your elbows high.

Bent Over Rows

This exercise has positive effects on your upper back, as well as the side of your back . If you find it challenging to do this exercise, you can consider sitting on a chair while performing it. If you are one of those people who might find the "bent over rows" too easy, you can make it heavier by using dumbbells.

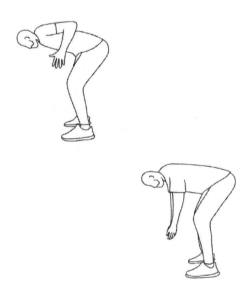

Do this exercise as follows:

1. Stand in such a way that your feet are hip-width apart, making sure that your toes are pointing forward.
2. Hinge at the hip so that your chest points down toward the floor, while your hips keep back. Your upper body should be slightly perpendicular to the lower body.
3. Keep a slight bend in the knees.
4. Start the exercise by hanging your hands straight down to the ground at around chest level or a bit below, as if you were picking up something.
5. Row your arms up to just under your chest and squeeze your shoulder blades while doing so. Repeat this movement while maintaining the same posture for the rest of your body.

Bent-Over Reverse Flies

As you perform this exercise, you should feel its effect on your upper back. If you do it more consistently, this workout is great for improving posture. In the event that you feel a bit overwhelmed by this exercise, sitting on a chair can help. If you want to add some weight to the exercise, go ahead and get some dumbbells—you will certainly like the experience!

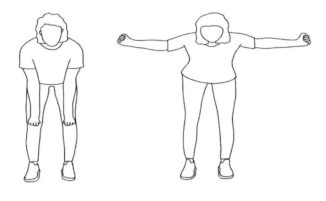

Here is how you can carry out the "bent over reverse flies":

1. Take a standing position, ensuring that there is a hip-distance between your feet. Your toes should be facing right ahead of you.
2. Bend forward so that your upper body is at a right angle with the lower part of your body. While in that position, bend your knees slightly.
3. Hang your arms straight down under your shoulders, with your palms open.
4. While keeping your arms straight, lift your arms straight out to the sides, until they reach the same height as the

bent upper body. Be sure to squeeze your shoulder blades together as you do so.

5. Bring the arms back to the hanging position and repeat this movement as described in (4) above.

W Raise

With the W-raise, you can build strength and muscle in your shoulders. This workout specifically targets muscles such as the upper and middle trapezius, as well as the posterior deltoids. It is possible to upscale this exercise by incorporating dumbbells.

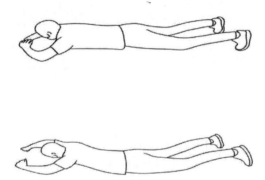

The procedure for this exercise is described below:

1. Lie down on your tummy. Lie down on your stomach with your legs straight out behind you on the floor. The

arms, slightly bent so that the lower arm points forward, should also be on the ground. Keep your head off the floor.

2. Lift your arms off the floor as much as you can, without changing the shape they assumed when they were still on the floor.

3. Place your arms back on the floor again and repeat. Please note that the goal is to form a W shape with your head and arms.

Chapter 6:

The Chest

After reading this chapter, you will be in a position to carry out simple chest exercises to help you with balance, reduction in joint pain, and enhanced fitness levels. You will also learn about the different muscles that you find in your chest. This chapter also provides tips on how you can intensify your exercises in order to get the most out of them. Let's get more details on how to stay fit in old age.

Your Chest and Exercises

You need to work your chest muscles in order to perform various functions throughout the day. In addition to improving your physique, working your chest muscles serves as a starting point for the many movements required for athletics and various exercises. It is important to note that for you to move your arms across the body, chest muscles are involved. Up and down movements that you do with your hands are also supported by chest muscles.

Other movements that require chest muscles include rotation, adduction, and flexion (Waehner, 2020). The most common chest exercises push your body away from the arms or the arms away from your body. As you do your chest exercises, bear in mind that particular exercises stimulate your chest in various ways. Stronger chest muscles also result in a body that is subsequently strong.

Common exercises, for instance, push-ups, make use of the chest muscles. Due to the fact that your chest muscles are large and can withstand more weight, it is possible for you to burn more calories when you involve them in your exercises. Actually, as you work your chest, you will also be involving your arms and shoulders. This allows you to simultaneously exercise many of your body parts, all in one go. Interestingly, for smaller muscle groups, a chest workout acts as a great way of warming up.

It is worth mentioning that as you do your chest exercises, many other organs are involved, for instance, the lungs. Keeping your lungs and chest wall mobile will help you go a long way in fighting some of the conditions that come with aging. Some of these conditions include asthma, emphysema, and chronic bronchitis (betterhealth, 2012).

Although it may be fun to go out and exercise, it is important to note that exercising comes with a lot of benefits, especially if you are a senior citizen. In Australia, it has been noted that approximately only one in ten people that are over 50 years old carry out sufficient exercises to realize any benefit when it comes to cardiovascular health (Better Health Channel, 2012). Estimates have also been put forward that approximately half of the physical deterioration linked to old age may be because of the lack of physical activity. If you are above the age of 60, consider the need for adequate fitness levels to assist you in recovering from illnesses, lowering your risk of disease, and most of all, maintaining your independence.

Numerous studies have alluded to the fact that it is never too late to get fit. No matter what age you are, please note that your body will respond to exercise. It is essential to start slowly, then increase the intensity of the exercise as you go. Always be in consultation with your doctor or physical trainer before you move to a more intense exercise. Consultation is also important when you want to increase the frequency with which you carry out your chest exercise or any in general.

Chest Muscles

The pectoralis muscle is the major component of the chest in relation to muscles. This muscle connects the bones of the upper arm and shoulder with the chest's front walls. The pectoralis muscle can be further broken down into major and minor muscles. In the human body, these two muscles are found on both sides of the breastbone, pectoralis major is dominant in the upper chest. On the other hand, the pectoralis minor is found under the major one. In the pectoral region, you will also find the subclavius and serratus anterior (Jones, 2021).

The Pectoralis Major Muscle

The pectoralis major is situated in the thoracic cage, on the front surface. In the gym, these muscles are commonly called the "pecs muscles." The origins of the pectoralis major are broad, such that it is broken down into three parts, namely, sternocostal, abdominal, and clavicular parts. These three parts go sideways to eventually join and attach to the humerus. The primary function of this entire muscle is to allow the arm's internal rotation and adduction on the shoulder joint. Adduction refers to the action of bringing something closer to a reference point. Independent action of the clavicular part assists to bend the extended arm up to the point of a right angle. The sternocostal part, on the other hand, helps to extend the flexed arm by a downward pulling action.

The pectoralis major is fan-shaped and consists of clavicular and sternal heads. The clavicle refers to the collarbone, while sternum is the breastbone (Augustyn, 2020). We mentioned earlier that the origins of the pectoralis major are broad. Let's break these down and get more information on the three sites that the muscle originates from. The clavicular part, as the name suggests, comes from the front surface of the clavicle's medial half. Coming from the sternum's front surface and costal cartilages' anterior aspects is the sternocostal part. Originating from the front layer of the rectus's sheath is the abdominal part. This is the smallest part of the pectoralis major muscle.

The pectoralis major muscle is housed in the anterior chest wall. In females, the muscle is covered by the breast, whereas in men, it is protected by subcutaneous tissue, a strong layer of fascia, as well as adjacent skin. It is also important to note that the greater part of the pectoralis major muscle protects the pectoralis minor, serratus anterior, and the upper six ribs' anterior surface. In between the clavicle, deltoid, and pectoralis major muscles is a triangular depression referred to as infraclavicular fossa. The triangular depression is also known as Mohrenheim's fossa (Grujičić, 2022). The pectoralis major is responsible for providing locomotion to each shoulder joint in a total of four different directions. Its other function is to keep your arms attached to your body.

The Pectoralis Minor

Situated under the pectoralis major is the pectoralis minor. It arises from the middle ribs such that it goes and attaches to the scapula. Specifically, the pectoralis minor has its origins in the third to fifth ribs. From here, that is where it arises to attach to the scapula. Another name for the scapula is the shoulder blade. Pectoralis minor helps to draw the shoulder in a forward and downward manner (Augustyn, 2020). Put in another way, the pectoralis minor helps to stabilize the scapula by drawing it antagonistically to the thoracic wall.

The Serratus Anterior

In the chest wall, you will find the serratus anterior, which serves to form the axilla region's medial border. The muscle is comprised of a number of strips that stem from the lateral aspects of eight ribs, from the first one to the eighth. These, in turn, insert onto the rib-facing surface of the scapula's medial border. The serratus anterior serves to rotate the scapula, thereby making it possible for the arm to be raised above 90 degrees. Its other function is to allow the scapula to be held against the ribcage.

The Subclavius

Underneath the clavicle is a tiny muscle that runs horizontally, called the subclavius. In case there is a clavicular fracture or any other trauma, the subclavius provides a shield to the nearby neurovascular structures. The subclavius's origins are on the first rib's junction and its costal cartilage. It arises to attach onto the inferior surface of the clavicle's middle third. The subclavius serves to depress and anchor the clavicle.

Exercises for Your Chest

There are a number of chest exercises that you can do to help with your health and fitness, especially when you are over 60 years of age. Some of the exercises include wall push-ups, floor press, and flies. Let's get more details on how to do each of these in this section. Please choose one chest exercise per workout.

Wall Push-ups

Wall push-ups tend to be a great option when it comes to reducing some of the strain that results from gravity. This makes it easy for you to carry it out if you are a senior citizen, yet it involves the physical training of your chest, shoulders, and back. Wall push-ups allow you to polish up your form, make you ready for standard push-ups, and help you strengthen your muscles. For senior citizens, wall push-ups help in starting slow so that an appropriate mind-body connection is developed while engaging the proper muscles for the task. In old age, you may be experiencing mild wrist, elbow, or lower back pain. Wall push-ups are for you if you are such a person. Although there are many variations to the push-up, the good news is that great benefits can be realized, even from the simple wall push-up. By performing this exercise, your posture is enhanced and your upper body is strengthened, thereby allowing you to experience improved function in your everyday life.

Before we get the instructions for carrying out wall push-ups, let's get some details on exactly which muscles are utilized when doing this exercise. The chest muscles, such as the pectoralis major and the pectoralis minor are involved during Wall push-ups. Deltoids, triceps, and the serratus anterior are also trained when you are doing Wall push-ups. The core muscles, for example, obliques, rectus abdominis, multifidus, and the transversus abdominis, together with the upper and lower back muscles such as the rhomboids, spinal stabilizers, and the trapezius are not left out when carrying out Wall push-ups. To a certain extent, Wall push-ups also involve your lower body muscles such as quads, glutes, and calves, which are important for stability (Davidson, 2021). In addition to other benefits, these muscles assist in the enhancement of your balance, upper body mobility, as well as postural stability.

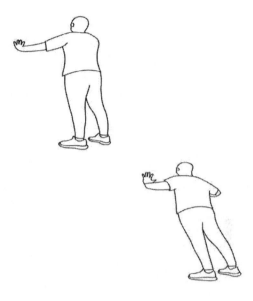

Now, to do a wall pushup, make sure you have a wall in front of you, and then follow these instructions:

1. Stand in front of the wall, at arm's length away from it. Ensure that your feet are hip-width apart.
2. Put both palms on the wall at shoulder height and shoulder-width apart.
3. Bend your elbows slowly and start to lean toward the wall up to a point at which your nose almost gets in contact with it. Make sure that your back keeps straight and the elbows are bending at approximately 45 degrees.
4. Slowly push back to where you started. Repeat several times. To make the exercise more challenging, increase your distance from the wall.

Floor Press

The floor press is a simple addition to your training plan. It targets the shoulders, triceps, and chest. When doing this exercise, be sure to keep your spine flat and avoid arching your lower back. Also, flare out your elbows so that you are able to target your pecs. In addition to that, keep your wrists in a neutral position.

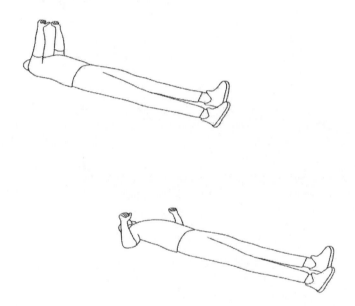

To do a floor press, here are the steps that you can follow:

1.   Lie with your back on the floor and make sure that your legs are extended and flat on the floor as well. Throughout the exercise, your head must be positioned on the floor.

2. As you start this exercise, make sure that your elbows are on the ground and your hands are pointed upwards, toward the ceiling, and at shoulder-width apart.
3. The next step is to press your hands over your chest so that they become fully stretched. Repeat these hand movements several times. Consider holding dumbbells in each hand in order to make the training more challenging.

Chest Flies

The chest flies will do you a good service when it comes to strengthening your shoulders and chest. The triceps are also worked when doing chest flies. Another remarkable benefit that you can get from performing chest flies is the increased range of motion, tightness reduction in the upper body, as well as the potential lowering of your upper back pain (Chertoff, 2019). By performing chest flies, your shoulder retraction is enhanced.

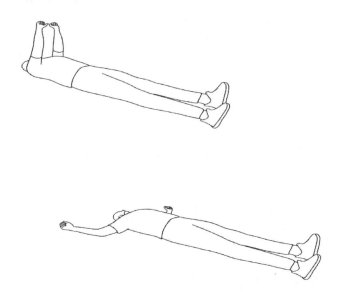

Here is the procedure for performing chest flies:

1. Lie flat on the floor facing upwards as you would when doing the floor press. Make sure that your back and head are positioned firmly on the floor throughout the movement.
2. Lift your arms above your chest so that they are outstretched. Clench your fists as if you are about to get into a fight.
3. Slightly bend your elbows as you lower your arms down to the sides. Lift them back up again to the initial position, making sure that your fists are facing each other. If you are doing it right, on your way down, it is normal to feel a slight stretch in your pecs.

4. Repeat this movement pattern. To make it more challenging and to get more benefits from this exercise, consider holding dumbbells in each of your hands.

Low Fly

The low fly targets the chest, though it also positively impacts the muscles of the shoulders and forearms. Like many other exercises, you can add some resistance by holding a pair of dumbbells as you perform it.

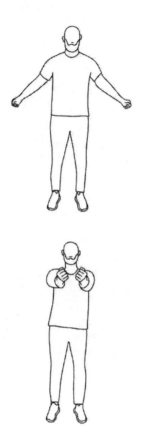

Here is how you can get this exercise done:

1. Stand so that your feet are facing forward and have a
    shoulder-width distance between them. With clenched
    fists, position your arms slightly behind you. There
    should be an approximated 45-degree angle between
    each arm and your torso.

2. Now, swing both arms to your front, keeping them straight all the way. Your hands should end up being parallel to each other at shoulder-height level in front of you.

3. Swing the arms back to the position in step 1 above and repeat step 2 again.

4. Keep repeating step 3 until the time allocated for this workout elapses.

Chapter 7:

The Shoulders

The main goal of this section is to help you to strengthen your shoulders through exercise. You might be wondering why we also focused on shoulders in a bid to keep you healthy as you age. There are a lot of changes to your shoulders that take place as you survive longer. One of the changes that are worth mentioning is that your shoulder range of motion reduces with age. Some findings report that men and women who are aged between 55 and 85 years of age experience a six-degree per decade reduction in shoulder range of motion (Purposed Physical Therapy, 2022). Such changes can significantly affect your daily activities more than you could probably imagine. The reduced range of motion can cause some pain when you are doing simple things like driving, carrying your groceries, tidying the house, passing food across the table, among other things.

Stronger shoulders are also more resistant to unnecessary and avoidable injuries. You won't need to worry about injuries when you play baseball with your grandkids during their weekend visits. Strong shoulders are also associated with more self-esteem. Here is an easy and relatable example. When shoulders are weak, they don't stay in position. Rather, they sort of fall down or droop. That posture, on its own, can come across as a negative thing when it comes to self-confidence. In addition to this, your confidence in doing things may be compromised because of the pain that is usually associated with shoulders that are weak.

Shoulder muscles ensure that the joint on your shoulder is stable. They also come in handy in enabling your hands to move in various directions. This, therefore, further explains why you need to exercise and keep your shoulders on point. Before we go on to the exercises that you can perform for your shoulders to become strong, we will discuss the muscles that are found in the shoulders.

Shoulder Muscles

The shoulder is one of those parts that are supported by a lot of muscles as you will see in this section. It has about 20 muscles (Hecht, 2020). This section has been dedicated to exploring the different muscles that are found in the shoulders. We will also discuss the functions of these muscles.

Largest Shoulder Muscles

Let's look at some of the largest muscles that are related to or located in the shoulders in this section.

- **Pectoralis major:** This large muscle assumes the shape of a fan. It originates from your collarbone stretching into your mid-chest. This muscle is connected to the breastbone. The pectoralis major is the muscle that makes it possible for you to rotate your arm forward. This muscle also contributes to depression of the arm.
- **Rhomboid major:** We discussed this muscle when we talked about back muscles. It also fits this section because it is connected to the shoulder blade, having stretched from the vertebrae.
- **Deltoid:** This large muscle with a triangular shape is the one that covers the joint where the upper part of your arm inserts into the shoulder socket. This joint is called the glenohumeral joint. Deltoid muscles make it

possible for you to move your arm sideways, forward, and backward.

- **Serratus anterior:** This muscle has three sections. Overall, stretches from the shoulder blade at one end and then attaches to the first eight ribs on the other. All the three sections of the serratus anterior muscle collaboratively lift the ribs, an action that enhances breathing.
- **Trapezius:** This muscle is quite wide. It is found along the back part of your neck, as well as your shoulders. The trapezius also goes down your spine. The upper fibers of the trapezius enhance the elevation and rotation of the scapula. It also makes it possible for you to extend the neck.

Rotator Cuff Muscles

Have you ever wondered what keeps your upper arm in its place? It is the rotator cuff muscles. We will delve deeper into each of these muscles that are found in the rotator cuff in this section. Take note of the fact that the rotator cuff is highly involved in promoting the different forms of movement that happen in the shoulder area. Let's discuss more on the four muscles that make this happen.

- **Teres minor:** This muscle is narrow in nature and is located on the lower side of the upper arm. The teres minor also helps to attach the upper arm to the shoulder blade. This muscle is also involved in making lateral rotation of the arm possible.
- **Supraspinatus:** Triangular in shape, this muscle is located at the back region of the shoulder blade. The supraspinatus plays a major role in initiating abduction. Not only that, but this muscle also depresses the humerus head so that it can withstand the pull from the deltoid. The muscle also promotes external rotation,

considering that this muscle and the tendons' movement from the posterior to the anterior is a bit oblique.

- **Subscapularis:** This triangular muscle is not only the largest but also the strongest among all the muscles that are part of the rotator cuff. You will find it stretching from the shoulder blade, at the front of your upper arm. The role of this muscle is to adduct and rotate the humerus internally.
- **Infraspinatus:** This muscle is located close to the supraspinatus and has a triangular outlook. The infraspinatus is attached to the backside of the shoulder blade.

Other Shoulder Muscles

There are more shoulder muscles that we can talk about. We will discuss these 'other' muscles in this section.

- **Biceps brachii:** This muscle is double-headed as it originates from two regions that are at the top of the shoulder blade. These two parts of the biceps brachii ultimately join together and attach as a single muscle at your elbow. The major role of this muscle is in promoting the forearm's outward rotation, in addition to flexion functionalities.
- **Pectoralis minor:** Located just under the pectoralis major, this muscle appears thin and flat. It is linked to the ribs on positions three, four, and five. The pectoralis minor has a number of functions and these include internal and downward rotation of the scapula. Other effects on the scapula as enhanced by the pectoralis minor include depression, stabilization, and abduction.
- **Triceps:** This long muscle is found on the back of your upper arm. The triceps reach the elbows, having started

from the shoulders. This muscle protects from the possible displacement of the humerus. It does so by holding the ball of the humerus in position during movement.

- **Latissimus dorsi:** The latissimus dorsi starts from the backbone and ends at the lower region off the shoulder blade.

Let's Get Active!

To help you to keep your shoulders healthy and active, this section provides a set of exercises that have been prepared for you. For the purpose of this book and the nine-minute exercising session, select one shoulder exercise as part of the whole session. You have the leverage to choose a different one in another session if you don't want your workout sessions to feel repetitive.

Lateral to Frontal Raise

In this exercise, you will be training both the frontal and lateral heads of the shoulder. You can reduce the difficulty level of the exercise by performing it while seated on a chair. It is also possible to upscale the difficulty level by using dumbbells to add an extra form of resistance to the workout.

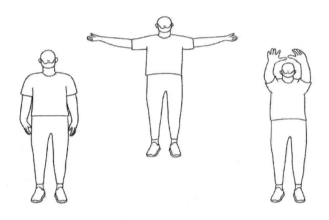

Here is the procedure for doing the lateral to frontal raise:

1. Stand with your feet together, while your arms hang at your side.
2. Keep your arms straight as you raise them out to the side all the way until your hands are at the same height as your shoulders.
3. From there, swing your arms slowly out in front of you while keeping them stretched out.
4. Return your arms back to the position that you ended up in during step 2.
5. Now, lower your arms back down to your sides again.
6. Repeat the movement that is described in steps 2 to 5.

Shoulder Press

The largest muscles in the shoulder are the main targets for this exercise. Like many other exercises that we described before, the level of difficulty for this exercise is adjustable. To upscale the exercise, add a pair of dumbbells to the regular procedure. To downscale it, get a chair and do the exercise while sitting.

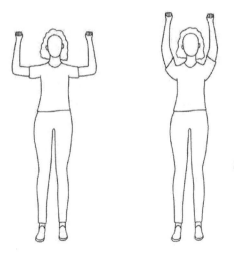

Workout your shoulders' largest muscles by following this procedure:

1. Stand with your feet at shoulder width and your toes facing forward.
2. Start with your hands bent at shoulder height just outside the shoulder width. Your palms should be facing toward the ceiling while the elbows point down. Hold your core tight throughout the movement.
3. From the position in step 2 above, stretch your arms over your head and bring them closer to each other until they almost touch at the top.
4. Return to the start position and repeat.

Rotator Cuff Rotation

This exercise helps to strengthen your rotator cuff. Sit down to downscale it or include a pair of dumbbells to upscale, depending on your needs and preferences. A key point that you should note is that your elbows should maintain their position throughout the movement. In other words, the rotation should occur only through the shoulder joint.

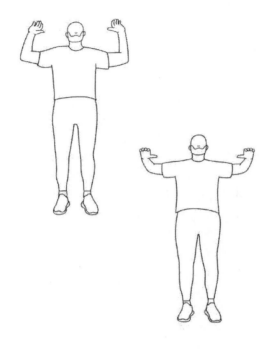

The exercise can be easily performed as follows:

1. Assume a standing position, making sure that there is a shoulder-width distance between your feet.
2. Stretch your arms straight out to your sides and up to shoulder height. Now, bend your lower arms so that they face forward. This means that you will form a 90-degree angle between your upper and lower arms. This is your start position.

3. Now, lift the lower arm so that it faces toward the ceiling or sky. While maintaining the 90-degree angle, reassume the start position.
4. Repeat the up and down rotations, making sure that the rest of your body does not move.

Around the World

The 180-degree movements of your hands during this exercise are great for your deltoids. The stimuli that this exercise produces for your lateral and front deltoids encourage the new growth of muscles. It is still fine if you feel that doing this exercise while sitting on a chair is better for you. However, if the exercise feels too light for you, get some dumbbells and get started.

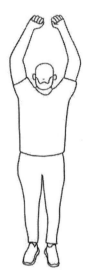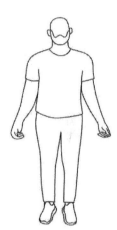

Get ready to follow these steps as you do the "around the world" exercise:

1. Stand, with your feet close to each other and facing forward. Keep your arms at your sides and clench your arms into fists. This marks your start position.
2. Now, simultaneously raise your hands sideways until they point up toward the ceiling or sky. Keep the fists clenched as you do so. Bring these fists as close to each

other as possible above your head but don't let them touch.

3. Bring the two arms down again to the position where they were when you started.
4. Repeat.

Shrugs

As simple as they might appear, shrugs are a great addition to your workout routine if you want stronger shoulders, upper back muscles, and neck. This exercise also contributes to an improved posture. One of the muscles that are targeted by shrugs is the trapezius. This helps to lower the possibility of overstraining the muscles on your shoulder and neck.

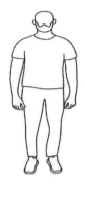

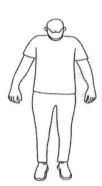

Here is how you can do this exercise:

1. Stand, with a shoulder-width distance between your feet. Relax your hands at your sides.
2. Raise your shoulders as high as you can and lower them again.
3. Repeat step 2 as many times as time allows you.

Chapter 8:

The Core

A healthy core significantly contributes to a vibrant, strong, and disease-free body overall. A stronger core plays a central role in enhancing good balance and mobility, without which you are more likely to incur injuries as a result of falls. As people grow older, wound-healing takes longer so you can't afford to have that happen to you if it can be avoided. When you have a strong and healthy core, the muscles of other parts of your body will put in less effort in helping you to complete your everyday tasks. The opposite is also true—the weaker the core, the harder the other body muscles would need to work for tasks to be completed.

In addition to aiding better balance, a stronger core also improves your coordination and posture. Your spine which is so much involved in giving you balance is also supported by the core, thereby making it function better. Better balance and stability usually correlates with increased confidence. A weaker core can make life quite unenjoyable. Even getting out of bed in the morning can become a challenge. To individuals who have a weak core, this usually comes with some pain. Exercising the muscles of the core is a great remedy for managing back pain. General body strength increases when your core is strong. Results from some scientific studies suggest that there is a 30% increase in body strength when seniors engage in core strengthening workouts (American Senior Communities, 2015).

Now that you have an understanding of what exercise can do for your core, this section will go on to discuss the different muscles that make up the core. The chapter will also end by giving you procedures for exercises that are effective in strengthening your core.

Core Muscles

Abdominal and back muscles make up the core. Spine, hip, and pelvic muscles are also involved. This section will delve a little deeper in highlighting the specific muscles that make your core play its various roles in the body.

- **Transverse abdominis:** This is also referred to as the transversus abdominis or the lower abs. This muscle is the deepest layer when we talk about abdominal muscles. The transverse muscle stretches from the ribs seven to twelve, ending at the pelvis. The primary function of this muscle is to keep your internal organs in place. Additionally, the transverse abdominis maintains the tension in the abdominal wall. This is of paramount importance as it keeps the pelvis and spine stable before, during, and after any form of movement.
- **External and internal obliques:** The abdominal wall has three layers and two of them are made up of oblique muscles while the third one is the transverse abdominis. The names of the internal and external obliques are derived from the location and shape of the muscles. Internal and external simply refer to inside and outside, respectively. Oblique refers to the slanting orientation of these muscles. These two muscles run on the sides of your core and they work together in their functions. The primary role of oblique muscles is stabilization. Both obliques can operate in a bilateral manner to flex the trunk, thereby compressing its

contents. Unilaterally, when these muscles flex the trunk, it moves to one side. So each oblique muscle would move the trunk toward one side while the other moves it to the opposite direction.

- **Multifidi:** The multifidi are found on each side of your spinal column. These muscles are the second of the three layers of t that make up the intrinsic layer of back muscles. Each of these muscles has a series of small bundles of muscles that are triangular. The multifidus muscle has four parts, which are, the cervical, thoracic, lumbar, and sacral. The cervical is your neck; the thoracic generally corresponds with the upper and mid-back region; the lumbar is the synonym for your lower back; the sacral corresponds to the region below your back. The multifidus muscles are unique and that is believed to give them more strength. This makes the core much stronger. When the multifidi contract, back extension results. These muscles maintain the stability of the spine during movement.

- **Erector spinae:** There are three main muscles that make up the erector spinae. These are the longissimus, iliocostalis, and spinalis. Please note that each of these main muscles of the erector spinae is further divided into three more muscles each, to make them nine more. The longissimus is further divided into longissimus capitis, longissimus cervicis, and longissimus thoracis. For iliocostalis, there is iliocostalis cervicis, iliocostalis thoracis, and iliocostalis lumborum. The spinalis divides into spinalis capitis, spinalis cervicis, and spinalis thoracis. All the erector spinae muscles are located along the spine. The primary function of the erector spinae is extending the spine.

- **Rectus abdominis:** Some refer to this muscle as the abs muscle. It is the one that forms the six-pack, which is quite visible in people with low contents of abdominal fat. The rectus abdominis stretches from the rib cage until it attaches to the pubic bone. The major role of this muscle in your body is to promote body movement between the rib cage and pelvis.

Work Out That Core!

Every human being is better off with a stronger and healthy core and you, as a senior citizen, are not an exception. Actually, a stronger core is even more important. This section is a compilation of exercises that will positively impact your core. Please note that you need to choose two exercises that target your core and incorporate them into your nine-minute session each time.

Elbow to Knee

This exercise works the side of your core, as well as the front. At the same time, it works on improving your balance. Please note that there is no harm in performing this exercise while seated on a chair if you feel that it is too difficult for you.

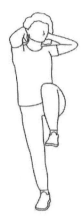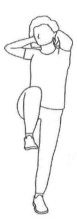

The step-by-step procedure for the "elbow to knee" exercise is as follows:

1. Stand with hip-width distance between your feet.
2. Raise your hands to the side of your head with your elbows pointing down toward the ground. This pose marks your start position.
3. Raise your right knee up as high as possible while simultaneously bringing down your left elbow. To do this well, assume that you are trying to reach your right knee with your left elbow, even though they might not touch.

4. Change sides. This time lift up your left knee while bringing down the right elbow.
5. Perform steps 3 and 4 repeatedly.

Russian Twist

When you perform the Russian twist, you will be doing a great favor to your core, spine, and obliques. Additionally, the Russian twist enhances your balance, thereby promoting better stability. If the exercise is too difficult, consider sitting on the front of a chair and leaning slightly back. In the event that the exercise is too easy, try lifting your feet off the floor when performing the exercise. This creates more instability and makes the exercise harder and more challenging.

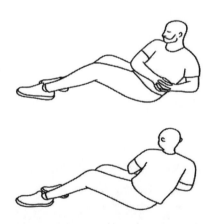

Here is how to do the Russian twist:

1. Sit on the ground with your feet out in front of you. You can use a mat or blanket for this exercise. Bring both of your knees up by bringing your feet closer to your body. Slightly lean backward with your upper body. Bring your arms in front of you, around your belly area, while clenching both hands together. This is your start position.

2. Swing the clenched hands to your sides, alternating between the right and left. So, you will be rotating your upper body and arms to one side and then the other.

3. Repeatedly perform step 2.

Standing Core Rotation

This exercise also has an amazingly positive impact on your core as it strengthens it. In its standard form, this exercise is performed while you are standing. However, you have the leverage to sit down if the standard version is a bit of a challenge for you.

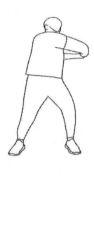
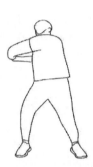

Performing this exercise is as easy as the following steps will show you:

1. Assume a standing position such that your feet are separated by hip-width distance. Bend slightly in your knees and bring your arms in front of you, form a circle with them, and hold the joined hands at shoulder height. This is the start position.

2. Rotate from the position described in 1 above toward your right side.

3. Swing back, past the original position, toward the left side.

4. Continue to repeat steps 2 and (3).

Lying Single Leg Lifts

This exercise has immense benefits on your core. Overall, it enhances your posture, balance, and strength for your everyday activities. If your back hurts while you're doing this exercise, try placing your hands under your butt for extra support.

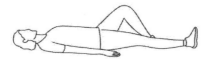

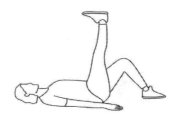

To complete this exercise, follow this procedure:

1. Lay with your back and allow your head to rest on the ground. A mat or blanket can help you to feel more

comfortable as you do this. Your legs should be parallel to the ground, while your feet face upward. Your hands should be on their respective sides. This position is your start pose.

2. Raise your right leg up in the air until the bottom of that leg's foot is pointing toward the ceiling. Make sure the left leg remains stuck to the floor as you do this.
3. Lower the raised leg back down to its original position.
4. With the right leg flat along the floor, lift the left one the same way you did in 2 above. Bring it down again.
5. Perform steps 2 to 4 repeatedly.

Crunches

Crunches can assist you in building muscle, in the same way, sit-ups do. However, the difference between sit-ups and crunches is that the latter specifically works on abdominal muscles only. This is the reason why individuals who want to build their six-pack abs will swear by it. Crunches also strengthen your core.

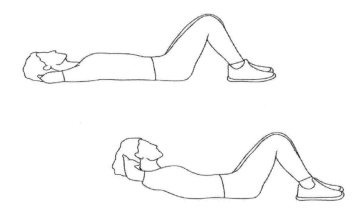

We have created a clear outline of how you can perform this exercise. Just follow this procedure:

1. Get your mat and lie down on your back. Lift your knees as much as is comfortable to you, making sure that your feet remain parallel to the floor and facing forward. You can open-up your knees a little bit to make the position more comfortable. Hold the back of your head with both palms. Right, you have just assumed your start pose.
2. Raise your head, shoulders, and chest area toward your knees as much as you can. Your hands should keep holding the back of your head. Also, be sure not to lift your lower back off the floor.

3. Place the raised part of your body back to its initial position.
4. Repeat steps 2 and 3.

Plank

The primary benefit of performing the plank exercise is to strengthen the core. This exercise has extra benefits as it also stabilizes your joints, in addition to amassing strength in both your upper and lower body. Holding a plank position will also enhance your flexibility, metabolism, posture, as well as balance, and coordination.

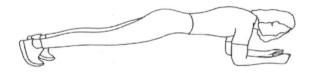

Here is how you can do this exercise:

1. Prepare your mat or blanket if you find doing the exercise directly on the floor uncomfortable.

2. Assume a crawling position and then let your lower arms lie parallel to the floor so that they carry the weight of your upper body. While in this position, glue your toes to the floor to keep your lower body up as well.

3. Hold this position for as long as possible. This is a more advanced movement, so don't be surprised if you can't hold it for the full 40 seconds. Focus on doing it as long as you can.

Chapter 9:

Nutritional Tips

Exercising and good nutritional habits work hand-in-hand in keeping you healthier and stronger. Together, these two can keep some common diseases at bay, which is a scenario that makes your old age more of a pleasure than a pain. Your risk of experiencing a heart attack, heart failure, and inflammation is reduced when you know what to feed your body with. Depression is also one of the things that you are less likely to worry about when your nutritional acumen is on-point.

Eating right is a great way of energizing your body in preparation for exercise sessions. Just remember not to eat immediately before you start your workout. Did you know that there are some foods that lighten up your mood? An individual with a better mood feels more driven to exercise and certainly, that is better than feeling like you are being forced to.In other words, when you know what to eat, it's also easier to incorporate exercise as part of your everyday lifestyle.

Knowing how important nutrition is to your health and fitness as a senior citizen, we have compiled this chapter to give you more insight on how to improve your eating patterns, in addition to what you should eat. We will also highlight some of the foods that you should stay away from and the reasons why this is so.

Your Food Checklist

Choosing the right food to eat has become quite difficult over the past few decades. This is attributed to the increased abundance and variety of foodstuffs. There is food everywhere and it sometimes makes sense if you get confused as to what to eat or avoid. Food is one of the commodities that are relatively affordable—you simply have to buy what you can afford. A bigger problem lies in the fact that most of the cheaper foods, especially in restaurants and other food outlets, are unhealthy if you consume them consistently. Even though you are living in such a world, you still need to eat healthily. For this reason, this section will discuss more the types of foods that you should never keep in your pantry or include in your grocery list. Not only that, but we will also give you ideas on what you should consider eating, depending on your preferences.

Foods to Avoid

In this section, we will look at some foods that you should try to avoid, as long as it's in your power to do so. The reasons why the foods that are highlighted in this section are not recommended differ for each food. To find out, set aside some time to go through this section.

Fried Foods

Fried foods are a danger to your health for three major reasons—they are usually high in calories, fats, and salt. High amounts of these are an easy way to attract diseases during your old age. When you eat fried foods as you age, you are simply taking in more calories than you can probably burn by living an active lifestyle. This is enhanced because sometimes, the intensity of your workouts might reduce as you grow older.

Fried foods are rich in what are called trans fats. These are a type of fat that elevates the levels of bad cholesterol in your body while reducing those of good cholesterol. Bad cholesterol is known as low-density lipoprotein (LDL) and it is associated with an increased risk of conditions such as heart diseases. Ideally, your body should have more good cholesterol, which is also called high-density lipoprotein (HDL).

High-temperature cooking such as frying sometimes results in the formation of a substance called acrylamide. This substance is toxic and is the product of a chemical reaction between sugars and asparagine, which is an amino acid. Fried potatoes, for example, have a significant amount of acrylamide. Some studies showed that the toxic acrylamide is implicated in certain types of cancer, including ovarian and kidney cancer (Friedman, 2003; Pelucchi et al., 2014).

Here, you should also take note of the fact that it might not be the actual ingredients or foods that are bad for you, but the cooking method. Instead of eating French fries, you can decide to boil your potatoes. The latter method is far more healthier than the former. If you eat 100 grams of French fries, you would have taken in around 320 calories, alongside 20 grams of fat. Now, consuming 100 grams of baked potato will see you eating 93 calories and no fat at all (McDonell, 2017).

Sugar-Sweetened Food and Drinks

Imagine hot weather where you are feeling thirsty to death. The greatest temptation you might face in such a scenario is feeling like grabbing a cold soft drink or any other drink with added sugar. Well, that is a mistake that you should train yourself to avoid because sugary drinks pose a danger to your health.

Imagine this—a 12-ounce serving of cola may harbor up to 39 grams of sugar. This is about 10 teaspoons of sugar, all in a drink.

Added sugar is also referred to as simple carbohydrates because it can be easily broken down by the body. Unlike the more complex carbohydrates like fiber, sugar is quickly broken down during digestion and floods your bloodstream in no time after eating. This means that there will be far more glucose in the blood than what your body can use. Please note each time you eat a sugary food and glucose is released into your bloodstream, your body will take the amount that it requires for important body processes such as respiration. A certain amount of the excess glucose remaining in your bloodstream will be stored in the liver and muscles, to prepare for emergent needs for energy sources in your body. If there is still more glucose in your bloodstream, your body has no choice other than to store this as fat.

Foods Rich in Added Fat

The reason why we are emphasizing 'added' fat is the fact that not all fats are bad in your diet. As a matter of fact, there are certain fats that you should include because your body needs them, too. Mind, even the cells of your body have lipids in their walls. You need fats but you need to know the right ones and the amounts to consume.

There are unsaturated and saturated fats. Unsaturated fats are the ones that are unlikely to cause harm to your body, as long as you eat amounts that are not excessive. Saturated fats are dangerous as far as your health is concerned. Unfortunately, saturated fats are the ones that are usually added to foods. As we mentioned before, saturated fats also increase the levels of LDL cholesterol in your body. Eating foods that have added fat will therefore cause unwanted weight gain, along with a myriad of other diseases.

Caffeinated Products

Apart from your coffee, you can also find caffeine in products such as other teas, chocolates, certain sodas, and some medications. When you take caffeine, your sleeping habits are negatively affected. Additionally, caffeine triggers anxiety. You become more prone to irregularities in the way your heart beats and this is not a good sign, especially if you had problems with your heart before.

Food to Eat

Are you feeling like all your favorite foods are being labeled as 'unhealthy'? Not to worry, there is still a lot that you can eat as you will find out in this section. There are many food types and ingredients out there that are prepared in a healthy manner to produce delicious meals that do not threaten your health.

High Fiber Foods

The main reason why whole foods are recommended for consumption is the fact that they are rich in fiber. In simple terms, fiber is a complex carbohydrate that cannot be digested. Fiber is classified as either soluble or insoluble, depending on its solubility in water. Foods that are rich in fiber include legumes like beans, fruits like apples, whole grains like wheat, and vegetables like broccoli.

There are a number of reasons why fiber-rich food is regarded as good for your body. Your digestive system harbors various types of bacteria, with up to a thousand species that are labeled as "good bacteria" (Gunners, 2018). These microorganisms improve the digestion process, making it more effective. The presence of good bacteria reduces the risk of inflammation of the gut. They also contribute to improving digestive disorders like irritable bowel syndrome (Scarpellini et al., 2007). More importantly, the survival of these good bacteria in your gut highly depends on the amount of fiber that you can provide for them to eat. Therefore, the more fiber you eat, the stronger your gut microflora will be.

Eating foods that are rich in fiber can also be a strategy for maintaining a good and healthy weight. Fiber stays longer in the digestive system after you have consumed it. This means that you will feel fuller for longer, a scenario that reduces the chances of snacking on unhealthy foods.

Some studies suggest that soluble fibers that are highly viscous can reduce your glycemic index (McRorie and McKeown, 2017). The term "glycemic index" refers to the number that measures the extent to which a carbohydrate food can increase glucose levels in the blood. Therefore, soluble and viscous fibers can control the amount of glucose that reaches your bloodstream after eating a meal that is carbohydrate-rich. This reduces the risk of diabetes as well. Fiber-rich foods also reduce the risk of constipation, and colorectal cancer (Kunzmann et al., 2015).

Vitamin D-Fortified Milk

When you buy your milk or milk alternatives, look for the ones that are labeled as "Vitamin D fortified." These products contain Vitamin D within them. Considering the many benefits that come with taking Vitamin D, drinking it in milk is one easy strategy for providing your body with enough of this nutrient. Please note that for all adults, the recommended daily intake of Vitamin D is 20 micrograms per day (Danahy, 2020). Vitamin

D can be easily absorbed from the sun but most lifestyles, as well as some seasons and climates, won't afford you the opportunity to get the nutrient that way. This makes Vitamin D a necessity, especially if you are a senior citizen.

Vitamin D is good for the development of healthy bones. Milk doesn't contain Vitamin D naturally, but it has calcium, which also contributes to stronger, healthier bones. Therefore, adding Vitamin D to milk makes a product that is excellent for bone health and maintenance. With the combination of calcium and Vitamin D, you prevent osteomalacia, which can affect older adults. Osteomalacia is a condition where your bones are too soft, a state that can lead to pain and instability.

Vitamin D also plays an important role in enhancing the proper growth of your cells. It also improves your muscle and nerve function. This nutrient also helps to promote a healthier immune system you really need this. If you take in vitamins, you are unlikely to deal with issues like inflammation, heart disease, some cancers, and also diabetes (National Institutes of Health, 2022).

Fluids

Every human body, whether young or old, is about 60% water (Sissons, 2020). This fact is partly explained by the fact that every process that takes place in your body requires water for it to be successful. The fluid that lubricates your joints also includes water. Respiration and other biochemical processes also need water for their progress. Water also aids the transportation of nutrients and digestion. For you to meet the water needs of your body, please heed the following recommendations (Schein, 2020):

- Drink 2500 milliliters of water per day if you are a man. This translates to about ten cups of water.

- Take about 2000 milliliters of water per day if you are a woman. This is approximately eight cups.

The differences in the amounts that are needed by men and women are due to the varying metabolic needs. As a matter of fact, the Basal Metabolic Rate (BMR) for men is higher than that of women. The BMR refers to the minimal amount of energy that your body requires for it to stay alive.

For some reason, seniors tend to naturally reduce their water intake as they age. This is mainly due to physiological changes in their bodies that they don't have much control over. Such changes include reduced thirst. This is why you need to devise strategies for making drinking water a habit, even when you don't feel like it.

Let's go into the nitty-gritty of why seniors need to drink more water:

- **Enhanced kidney function:** As you age, the efficiency of your kidneys tends to reduce. Kidneys are highly involved in maintaining a balance of fluid levels. They filter wastes from the blood, among other crucial functions. Drinking more water keeps kidney function at its peak.
- **Avoiding urinary tract infections:** Visiting the bathroom more often can be boring, especially when movement is also difficult. Since urinary incontinence is a common issue among seniors, most of them end up reducing their fluid intake to control it. This intervention is not good as it can lead to other urinary tract infections.
- **Maintaining optimum brain function:** Dehydration also hinders the proper functioning of your brain. Drinking enough water contributes to better brain functionalities, including memory and other cognitive abilities.

How can you improve your water intake, considering that even the physiological changes in your body seem to be supportive of low water intake? There are various strategies that might be of help and they include the following:

- **Set a reminder:** It's easy to forget to drink water when you are not necessarily feeling thirsty. Setting reminders for drinking water might help. Just train yourself to obey the reminders.
- Eat fruits and vegetables: Some fruits and vegetables contain remarkable amounts of water so eating them can be a great way for sneaking water into your body. It won't feel the same as directly taking a glass of water anyway. Fruits and vegetables like watermelons, pineapple, cucumbers, lettuce, and berries are good examples that you can eat for their water content.

- **Eat favorite meals and snacks that contain water:** Prepare your favorite smoothies and juices. You can even spice it up a bit by adding flavors to your water.

Diet and Healthy Weight

Good nutritional practices are an awesome way for maintaining a healthy weight, especially as you age. The quality of food that you consume determines the number of unuseful calories that will accumulate in your body. For example, a large intake of saturated fats will increase the amount of bad cholesterol in your body. Too much added sugar will end up being converted to fat for storage. The more this happens, the more you gain weight to unhealthy levels. Eat more of the foods that have been recommended in this book. That, together with the nine-minute workout, will keep unwanted extra calories at bay.

Weight and Diseases

By keeping a healthy weight, you will be doing yourself and your loved ones a favor. They will have you stick around for longer. This is because maintaining a healthy weight is a great strategy for keeping some diseases at bay. In this section, we will discuss some of the conditions that you can potentially avoid by eating well and maintaining a healthy weight.

Diabetes

Being overweight increases your risk of becoming diabetic. This is a disease that is caused by high amounts of blood sugar, which is also known as glucose. At any given period, there are certain amounts of blood sugar that your body can tolerate. Glucose levels that exceed these will cause diabetes. Insulin, the hormone that regulates the amount of glucose in your blood might become ineffective in the presence of too much glucose in your blood. Diabetes can later develop into other conditions such as cataracts and you certainly want to avoid such instances.

Heart Disease

As you add more weight, some fat might also accumulate in vessels that carry your blood to and from different parts of the body. The more the fatty residues accumulate, the more difficult it becomes for the blood to move along the vessels with normal pressure. The lumen of the blood vessels reduces, thereby increasing the pressure at which blood passes through the arteries and veins. Such increased pressure may also damage arterial walls, which may cause leakages in the long run. Besides, your heart will need to pump harder to supply your body with oxygen dissolved in the blood. Waste removal from body cells is also impeded by this situation. With all such things going on, you risk being a patient of heart disease and other heart-related discrepancies like high blood pressure and atherosclerosis. These diseases are a threat to your lifespan so you should do the best that you can to maintain a healthy weight.

Sleep Apnea

Sleep apnea is a sleeping disorder that is characterized by discontinuous breathing patterns. Other common symptoms of this condition are feeling tired even after a long and deep sleep, as well as making loud snoring sounds. Although there are other factors, like smoking and nasal congestion that can cause sleep apnea, excess weight is one of the most common ones. A heart complication can also trigger sleep apnea over time.

There are three major types of sleep apnea that exist. These are:

- **Obstructive sleep apnea:** This is the most common type. It takes place when the muscles on your throat relax, thereby narrowing the air passages
- **Central sleep apnea:** This condition is due to the brain's failure to send the right signals to the muscles that are involved with regulating breathing processes.
- **Complex sleep apnea syndrome:** In this case, the patient has both obstructive and central apnea. This explains why it is labeled as 'complex' and as a syndrome. This type of sleep apnea requires immediate treatment attention as it can be so severe.

By working out and taking control of your dietary patterns, you lower the probability of being overweight. This is a step forward in also protecting yourself from conditions like sleep apnea.

Ischemic Stroke

An ischemic stroke emanates from faulty blood supplies to the brain or some parts of the organ. We explained how fatty deposits in blood vessels can reduce the supply of blood to different parts of the body where it should supply oxygen. When the blood reaches the brain at a rate that is too low to meet the oxygen and nutrient demands of this important organ, this might result in the death of the brain cells that are affected. This is how strokes come to be. The bottom line is that the inadequate supply of oxygen and nutrients to the brain is a result of unhealthy weight. The best part is that this is avoidable through eating healthy and following a consistent workout routine.

It is important to note that if you notice any signs or symptoms of a stroke, immediately approach a health professional and get some medical assistance. Here is just a quick heads-up to what you should be on the lookout for in order to quickly determine the possibility of a stroke:

- **Extreme headache:** A headache that is accompanied by dizziness and vomiting might be a sign of a possible stroke.
- **Confusion:** A stroke can cause confusion and difficulty in deriving meanings in conversations.

- **Numbness of the face, arm, and leg on one side:** The affected side of the brain might also affect parts on the same side as itself. You won't be able to use the hand or leg that is affected.
- **Optical discrepancies:** Strokes can affect your vision. You might fail to see things clearly or even see images in doubles.

How Much Should I Eat?

There are no "one-size-fits-all" stipulations with regard to how much you should eat. This is because there are various factors that affect the amount of food that you should eat. These include gender, body size, age, and activity levels.

Generally, men eat more than women because their nutritional needs are also higher. One of the explanations for this is that the overall height and weight of men are larger when compared to those of women. As a result of all this, men's calorie requirements surpass those of women. However, even among individuals of the same gender, nutritional and calorie needs may vary. For you to know your nutritional and calorie requirements, you can use calorie calculators that are available online. With these calculators, you can find out how many calories you need to eat each day.

Tips and Tricks for Avoiding Overeating

Do you find overeating inevitable and difficult to do away with? If yes, then this section is for you. Sometimes, unhealthy eating is not all about the types of foods that you eat, but the number of certain food items. This section provides a list of ideas that can help you to steer clear of overeating.

- **Develop the habit of eating one portion:** When you are eating at home, train yourself to eat one portion and stop when you feel satiated. The same applies when you eat out in restaurants. These food outlets usually serve more than one portion. Don't eat all of it—it's not a 'must.' Eat what is reasonably enough and carry the rest of the food home so that you can eat later or share with others. If you don't feel like taking the leftover food home, how about inviting a friend to eat it with you.

This helps to reduce the temptation to eat more than you should.

- **Stay away from screens when you are eating:** Keeping your eyes glued to a television, laptop, phone, or any other screen as you eat can cause overeating. Your focus will be derailed so you lose track of what you have eaten and might keep consuming food even after you are full.
- **Slow down when eating:** When you eat too fast, it becomes difficult to determine your satiation point. There is an increased probability of swallowing the air when you eat fast. This can even cause bloating. In one study that focused on children, the results showed that 60% of the participants who ate fast also ate more than they should (Lee et al., 2011). Eating and drinking slowly also allows you to enjoy the taste and flavors of what you are consuming.

- **Read nutritional facts on labels:** If you check the labels on foods that you buy, you will find information about the calorie content, as well as the nutrients and their relative amounts. Reading such information can enlighten on what you will be consuming should you choose to buy the food product. If some major nutrients are given in grams, you can translate them into calories using the following information: one gram of protein and carbohydrates translates to four calories each, while one gram of fat is equal to nine calories.
- **Plan ahead:** Whenever you have the energy and time to cook, do so and store the healthy food in the fridge. These foodstuffs might come in handy when you are unable to cook for any reason. This way, you won't have to eat unhealthy foods. You can also store frozen beans and vegetables that have a low sodium content. These can be quick add-ons to your meals. Canned fruits that are packed in juice or frozen fruits can come in handy when you need snacks.

- **Engage local food delivery programs:** Identify food delivery programs that are reliable and engage them to deliver your healthy ordered food when you are not in a position to cook.
- **Invite some company:** Invite a friend, colleague, or relatives to share your healthy meals with you. Lightly converse as you eat to reduce the speed at which you eat.
- **Eat all meals:** Skipping meals can cause you to feel excessively hungry. The result of this is possible overeating in a bid to deal with hunger.

Important Nutrients as You Age

Not all nutrients are equally vital to the body of a senior citizen. Knowing the nutrients that matter most will go a long way in helping you choose the right foods, for a healthier body. We will explore such nutrients in this section.

Proteins

Your diet should be rich in proteins as they significantly contribute to the health of your muscles. Excess consumption of proteins is great for preventing sarcopenia. This is a condition where skeletal muscle mass and strength are gradually lost. In addition to these benefits, protein also helps to manage your weight as well as keep balanced energy levels. Proteins are broken into amino acids in the body. These amino acids are then used by your body as necessary. Leucine is an amino acid that stimulates the synthesis of proteins in muscles (Baum et al., 2016). Turkey, chicken, eggs, and legumes are good sources of proteins.

Vitamins

Here are some of the "must-have" vitamins as a senior adult:

- **Vitamin A:** This vitamin improves your eyesight and immune system. Some of the sources of Vitamin A are eggs, liver, cheese, squash, carrots, and broccoli.
- **Vitamin C:** With adequate consumption of Vitamin C, you will heal faster when you are wounded. This vitamin also improves the efficacy of your immune system. Vitamin C is also involved in repairing tissues. You can get Vitamin C when you eat green peppers, citrus fruits, pineapples, berries, and tomatoes.
- **Vitamin B12:** Vitamin B12 has two major functions in your body. First, it takes part in the formation of your genetic material. Second, this vitamin contributes to the health of blood and nerve cells. Milk, red meat, yogurt, poultry, beef liver, and eggs are some of the excellent sources of Vitamin B12.
- **Vitamin D:** Vitamin D does good to your bones by maintaining your bone mass. This vitamin also positively affects your immune system. To get Vitamin D, directly expose yourself to the sun, as well as eat fortified dairy products and fatty fish.

Minerals

Your body will also need minerals like the ones that are listed in this section:

- **Calcium:** Calcium works together with Vitamin D in promoting healthy bones and teeth. Adequate intake of calcium lowers the probability of suffering from colon cancer, osteoporosis, and high blood pressure. Spinach, salmon, dairy products, kale, and dried beans contain high amounts of calcium.

- **Potassium:** Potassium reduces the risk of hypertension and kidney stones. This mineral also helps to maintain bone mass. To get your potassium, eat broccoli, bananas, avocados, yogurt, strawberries, and low-fat milk.
- **Iron:** Iron is part of the haem that makes hemoglobin, the molecule that transports oxygen to your muscles. Eating fruits that are rich in Vitamin C improves the absorption of iron. Some foods that are great sources of iron are eggs, red meat, poultry, tuna, and fortified cereals.
- **Zinc:** Zinc has positive effects on your immune system, thereby improving its efficacy. Most processes that take place in your body are enhanced by proteins that are called enzymes. Zinc is sometimes part of these enzymes. Eat food like oysters, beans, red meat, poultry, and whole grains for zinc.

Chapter 10:

Cardiovascular Training

Reading this chapter will equip you with knowledge on cardiovascular training for seniors. You will find out why it is good for you to perform aerobic exercises. This chapter will also give you some pieces of advice should you decide to start certain exercise routines or intensify the old ones that you have been doing before. The recommended amount of aerobic training is also included in this chapter. Let's get more details.

The Importance of Cardiovascular Training

If you are a senior, it is important to regularly carry out exercises so that you can delay the effects of aging on your body. As much as exercising is important, it is essential, though, to choose the right type of exercise to do depending on your physical capabilities. Although carrying out exercises is beneficial, please bear in mind that for seniors, some intense exercises may cause the development of cardiovascular risks.

Generally for senior citizens, the exercise intensity shouldn't be too high. Prior to planning a workout regime for seniors, it is essential to take note of any possible health risks and put them into consideration.

Aerobic Exercises

Aerobic exercises function in such a way that they pump oxygenated blood from the heart to other parts of the body, where it is needed. Aerobic exercises are responsible for stimulating the heart and breathing rates in order to maintain the rates per minute for long periods. Some of the exercises that you can carry out as a senior citizen include jogging or running, brisk walking, cycling, or gardening. Swimming is one other exceptional option that you can try. It is especially helpful if you are a senior with knee pain.

Benefits of Aerobic Exercises

Aerobic exercises are also known as cardio workouts, and they enhance the circulation of blood in the body. Cardio training assists in combating illnesses as well as cardiovascular conditions. According to the Lung Institute, an estimated 4.7 million adults are diagnosed with emphysema, while 10 million with chronic bronchitis (Medical Guardian, 2016). Living with these conditions can reduce your efficiency, but with an appropriate fitness routine, your health can be revived. Let's discuss more on the benefits of aerobic exercises for seniors.

Reduction of Blood Pressure

Cardio workouts raise the high-density lipoproteins (HDL) and lower the low-density lipoproteins in your blood. As such, the effect is that your blood pressure is remarkably lowered.

Improvement of Sleep

In old age, you may experience insomnia as well as other sleep disorders. It is important to note that aerobic exercises such as cycling and swimming help seniors in sleep improvement. Make sure to exercise at least two hours prior to your bedtime. Always complete your exercise approximately two hours prior to your bedtime.

Enhancement of Cardiovascular Health

Aerobic training is very effective if you are a senior who wishes to avoid cardiovascular conditions. Even for seniors who have experienced some cardiovascular conditions, it is helpful for them to carry out low-intensity exercises such as walking. Although walking may seem to be simple, please bear in mind that the exercise will go a long way in significantly improving your heart as well as its muscles.

Reduction of the Effects of Asthma

If you are elderly with asthma or breathing difficulty, you are recommended to do low-intensity cardio training. It is vital, though, to consult your doctor if you need to know about which physical training to do if you have asthma. This is because regular aerobics and physical training for asthmatics differ completely (Athulya admin, 2020).

In addition to the above-mentioned benefits, cardio training reduces the frequently occurring chronic pain in seniors. Furthermore, aerobic exercises assist in healthy weight management, improvement of cognitive and brain health, and enhancement of immunity. Overall, due to the cardio training, the quality of living is greatly improved.

The Recommended Amount of Cardio for Seniors

For any exercise, consistency is vital if you are to get the best results. In order for consistency to be possible, it helps a lot for the workout to be enjoyable. The more enjoyable it is, the easier it is to get done. It is, therefore, important to find out which exercise is enjoyable for you, so that your workout regime is centered around that.

The President's Council on Fitness suggests a weekly recommendation of 150 minutes for seniors to carry out aerobic training (Medical Guardian, 2016). Depending on your preferences, this recommendation can break down to the desired combination, just as long as you reach your 150-minute goal. For instance, the combination can be two 12-minute bursts of cardio, for seven days. It can also be three times a week, 50 minutes worth of exercise. However, for you to get the desired pulmonary benefits, you should perform anaerobic training for at least 10 minutes.

The Different Types of Cardio Training

Cardio training comes in many different forms. This may be a simple walk, jog, run, or sometimes ballroom dancing. Recently, there has been the introduction of a combination of sports that are merged to form one, thereby giving seniors an opportunity to enjoy and exercise, simultaneously. Let's get some more information on the types of cardio exercises that are available.

Jogging or Running

A quick jog or run early in the morning will do you good when it comes to aerobic training. Your heart rate and blood flow will increase, thereby creating a conducive environment for you to reap your cardio benefits.

Racewalking and Brisk Walking

Running a marathon may not sound like something you can manage. However, there are other things you could try, for example, racewalking. This functions similarly to a regular race, except for the fact that power walks are involved in place of runs. Racewalking offers you the opportunity to get competitive but without putting an excessive strain on yourself.

As compared to jogging, brisk walking is less intense. However, it is a good exercise to get your muscles working and your heart rate up. Brisk walking exerts less impact on your joints, especially if you have weak ankles or knees. In comparison with normal walking, brisk walking helps you improve your pace. This exercise also helps you when it comes to maintaining a good posture. For you to achieve maximum benefits through brisk walking, set your shoulders back and make sure that your back is held straight.

Cycling

Cycling is another great way to train cardio. After cycling for a few minutes, your legs will have undergone enough training to get your blood pumping. With this type of training, your heart and breathing rates will go up in no time. This allows you to reap the benefits of cardio training such as healthy lungs, increased immunity, and reduction of joint pains.

Rowing

Rowing is a team-based sport and another great form of cardio. If you want to undergo the experience of rowing but without the water, you can easily go ahead and try the rowing machine. This allows you to get the needed experience but without the use of a boat (Hegg, 2018).

Although the above-mentioned exercises are helpful in the health of seniors, they may be difficult to incorporate into their daily routines. There are other exercises that can be used to stimulate similar effects obtained from the usual jog or run. The added advantage of such activities is that they are enjoyable. Examples of activities that can be incorporated by seniors into their routine aerobic exercises include water aerobics, Ballroom dancing, swimming laps, and pickleball. Let's discuss each of these in greater detail in this section.

Water Aerobics

Performing cardio training in water is advantageous in that it is easier on your joints and muscles. When you shift your cardio training to the pool, your workout becomes low impact and still gives you greater resistance in comparison to when you are on dry land.

Ballroom Dancing

Over the past few years, Ballroom dancing has become a common activity for seniors. Dancing regularly provides you with remarkable cardio benefits. Furthermore, your cognitive skills are sharpened when you get to learn new dance moves. Other advantages include the improvement of coordination and balance, not forgetting the positive social component that the exercise will have on seniors.

Swimming Laps

Some people prefer hanging out in large groups of people whereas others enjoy their alone time. Swimming laps are perfect for you if you are a senior citizen who does not like group activities. This cardio training is excellent for your lungs. In addition to that, swimming laps will also have a positive impact on your cardiovascular health. By involving swimming laps into your routine, your endurance is built and your muscle strength is increased as well.

Pickleball

This is a new sport that suitably fits into the senior's aerobic exercises. It is a combination of wiffle ball, tennis, and badminton. It is good for people living with arthritis because the sport involves a racquet that is larger than the normal one. Their joints and bones undergo less strain because the court is smaller. Pickleball will help you enhance your balance and agility.

It is important to note that you can perform some cardiovascular exercises after a nine-minute exercise session if you still have the energy. Another strategy for incorporating cardiovascular exercises in your workout routines is by allocating to other days of the week when you are not doing the nine-minute workout in this book. In its natural setup, this workout program has some aspect of cardiovascular action incorporated in it. Remember, the rest period between each workout procedure is 20 seconds. This rest period is so short that the blood flow will still be high and the heart will still be pumping at a faster rate, by the time you start the next exercise. Simply put, the nine-minute workout is fully-packed.

Conclusion

Growing older is a natural process that cannot be avoided. However, you can make it enjoyable by looking after your well-being as you age. Most of the effects of natural aging processes take their toll as senior citizens adopt more sedentary lifestyles in their old age. The pain, fatigue, muscle loss, bone mass loss, and diseases that are associated with aging can be countered by taking measures such as exercising and eating a healthy, balanced diet. This way, older individuals will enjoy more balance, strength, and resilience.

This book introduces a nine-minute workout session that senior citizens can use to keep themselves fit. Before each workout session, it is recommended to take time to do the warm-up exercises that will prepare you for the main session. Warming up will gradually heat your body, thereby increasing your breathing and heart rate. This protects your body from the shock that it would otherwise experience if you were to start with the main workout. Please note that the warm-ups are not included in the nine minutes of working out.

For each region of the body that was targeted by the workouts, we explored the muscles that are found there, as well as their functions. This is to help you understand what is happening in your body as you work out. Each exercise in the set should be done for 40 seconds, separated by 20-second rest periods. In each nine-minute workout session, you will do leg, back, chest, shoulders, and core exercises. You will select a few exercises as instructed in the book for each region of the body. Some of the examples of exercises that are involved are as follows:

- **Leg exercises:** Superman, good mornings, lunges, air squats, and lying hip thrusts.

- **Back exercises:** W-raise, reach and pull, and bent over rows.
- **Chest exercises:** Floor press, wall push-ups, low fly, and flies.
- **Shoulder exercises:** Shoulder press, shrugs, and the lateral to frontal raise.
- **Core exercises:** Elbow to knee, standing core rotation, crunches, and Russian twist.

We also recommend that seniors include cardiovascular exercises in their workouts. These exercises like jogging, pickleball, and water aerobics can be done at the end of the nine-minute exercise that is presented in this book. The nine-minute workout itself has some aspects of cardiovascular activity, considering that it involves only 20 seconds of rest between different exercises. The heart rate will still be high by the time you start the next exercise.

This book also acknowledges the collaboration between diet and exercise in promoting a healthy body that is devoid of avoidable diseases. For this reason, we also explored how diet affects your health. Tips for avoiding overeating were also highlighted, including slowing down when eating and avoiding screens during meals. Proteins were emphasized as one of the most important macronutrients in older adults. Vitamins such as Vitamin A, C, D, and B12, as well as minerals like iron, zinc, and calcium, were also highlighted as necessities as individuals age.

With this nine-minute workout handbook, it is my desire that you become stronger and healthier. You will get the best results if you do the exercises consistently. Once you have witnessed your desired results, please tell a friend to tell a friend, so that we can save as many senior citizens as possible from misery in their old age. Happy training!

References

admin. (2020, March 25). *Aerobic exercises for seniors. Benefits of cardio workouts.* Athulya. https://www.athulyaliving.com/blogs/aerobic-exercises-for-seniors-everything-you-should-know.php

American Lung Association. (2020, July 13). *Exercise and lung health.* www.lung.org. https://www.lung.org/lung-health-diseases/wellness/exercise-and-lung-health

American Senior Communities. (2015, December 8). *The best core exercises for seniors.* Senior Living Communities and Nursing Homes in Indiana | ASC. https://www.asccare.com/the-best-core-exercises-for-seniors/

Asher, A. (2020, October 23). *Why is the multifidus muscle special?* Verywell Health. https://www.verywellhealth.com/multifidus-muscle-296470

Augustyn, A. (2020, March 12). *Pectoralis muscle: Definition, location, function, and facts.* Encyclopedia Britannica. https://www.britannica.com/science/pectoralis-muscle

Behm, D. G., Blazevich, A. J., Kay, A. D., & McHugh, M. (2016). Acute effects of muscle stretching on physical performance, range of motion, and injury incidence in healthy active individuals: a systematic review. *Applied Physiology, Nutrition, and Metabolism = Physiologie Appliquee, Nutrition et Metabolisme, 41*(1), 1–11. https://doi.org/10.1139/apnm-2015-0235

Benefits of dynamic stretching. (2015, December 10). New England Baptist Hospital. https://www.nebh.org/blog/benefits-of-dynamic-stretching/

Better Health Channel. (2012). *Physical activity for seniors.* vic.gov.au. https://www.betterhealth.vic.gov.au/health/healthylivi ng/physical-activity-for-seniors

betterhealth. (2012). *Breathing problems and exercise.* vic.gov.au. https://www.betterhealth.vic.gov.au/health/HealthyLi ving/breathing-problems-and-exercise

Chertoff, J. (2019, November 22). *Dumbbell chest fly: How to, benefits, safety, variations.* Healthline. https://www.healthline.com/health/exercise-fitness/dumbbell-chest-fly

Cleveland Clinic. (n.d.). *Leg Muscles: Anatomy and function.* Cleveland Clinic. https://my.clevelandclinic.org/health/body/22220-leg-muscles

Cordier, A. (2018, February 9). *5 reasons why warm up exercises are important.* Fitathletic.com. https://fitathletic.com/5-reasons-warm-exercises-important/

Csatari, J. (2021, March 5). *Weight loss, nutrition tips and recipes.* Eat This Not That. https://www.eatthis.com/

Danahy, A. (2020, February 21). *Vitamin D milk: Everything you need to know.* Healthline. https://www.healthline.com/nutrition/vitamin-d-milk

Davidson, K., & Davis, N. (2021a, December 6). *Wall push-ups: How to Do This Modified Pushup Variation.* Healthline. https://www.healthline.com/health/fitness-exercise/wall-push-ups

Davidson, K., & Davis, N. (2021b, December 6). *Wall push-ups: How to do this modified pushup variation.* Healthline.

https://www.healthline.com/health/fitness-exercise/wall-push-ups

Ellerton, H. (2018, January 29). *Static stretching versus dynamic stretching: Which is the best?* Human Kinetics Blog. https://humankinetics.me/2018/01/29/static-stretching-vs-dynamic-stretching/

Exercise mat – how to choose the best? (2019, February 10). Apus Sports. https://apus-sports.com/exercise-mat-how-to-choose-the-best/

Exploring the erector spinae muscles. 3D Muscle Lab. (2020, April 27). https://3dmusclelab.com/erector-spinae-muscles/

External and internal oblique muscles. (2018, January 9). Yoganatomy. https://www.yoganatomy.com/external-and-internal-oblique-muscles/

Friedman, M. (2003). Chemistry, biochemistry, and safety of acrylamide. A Review. *Journal of Agricultural and Food Chemistry*, *51*(16), 4504–4526. https://doi.org/10.1021/jf030204+

Grujicic, R. (2022, February 16). *Pectoralis major muscle.* Kenhub. https://www.kenhub.com/en/library/anatomy/major-pectoralis-muscle

Gunners, K. (2018, May 23). *Why is fiber good for you? The crunchy truth.*Healthline. https://www.healthline.com/nutrition/why-is-fiber-good-for-you

Healthline Editorial Team. (2018, January 21). *Chest muscles anatomy, diagram and function.* Healthline. https://www.healthline.com/human-body-maps/chest-muscles#1

Hecht, M. (2020, April 17). *Shoulder muscles: anatomy, function, and more.* Healthline. https://www.healthline.com/health/shoulder-muscles

Hegg, J. (2018, October 6). *50 Cardio exercises for seniors.* Vive Health. https://www.vivehealth.com/blogs/resources/cardio-exercises-for-seniors

Henwood, T. R., Riek, S., & Taaffe, D. R. (2008). Strength versus muscle power-specific resistance training in community-dwelling older adults. *The Journals of Gerontology: Series A, 63*(1), 83–91. https://doi.org/10.1093/gerona/63.1.83

Johns Hopkins Medicine. (n.d.). *Osteoporosis: What you need to know as you age.* www.hopkinsmedicine.org. https://www.hopkinsmedicine.org/health/conditions-and-diseases/osteoporosis/osteoporosis-what-you-need-to-know-as-you-age

Jones, O. (2021, October 15). *Muscles of the pectoral region.* TeachMeAnatomy. https://teachmeanatomy.info/upper-limb/muscles/pectoral-region/

Kahraman, T., Çekok, F. K., Üğüt, B. O., Keskinoğlu, P., & Genç, A. (2019). One-year change in the physical functioning of older people according to the international classification of functioning domains. *Journal of Geriatric Physical Therapy, 44*(1), E9–E17. https://doi.org/10.1519/jpt.0000000000000234

Kunzmann, A. T., Coleman, H. G., Huang, W.-Y., Kitahara, C. M., Cantwell, M. M., & Berndt, S. I. (2015). Dietary fiber intake and risk of colorectal cancer and incident and recurrent adenoma in the Prostate, Lung, Colorectal, and Ovarian Cancer Screening Trial. *The American Journal of Clinical Nutrition, 102*(4), 881–890. https://doi.org/10.3945/ajcn.115.113282

Louw, M. (2017, October 31). *Static stretching is safe before exercise.* Sports Injury Physio. https://www.sports-injury-physio.com/post/static-stretches-before-exercise

Mayo Clinic Staff. (2016). *The right way to warm up and cool down.* Mayo Clinic. https://www.mayoclinic.org/healthy-lifestyle/fitness/in-depth/exercise/art-20045517

McDonell, K. (2017, November 19). *Why are fried foods bad for you?* Healthline. https://www.healthline.com/nutrition/why-fried-foods-are-bad

McRorie, J. W., & McKeown, N. M. (2017). understanding the physics of functional fibers in the gastrointestinal tract: An evidence-based approach to resolving enduring misconceptions about insoluble and soluble fiber. *Journal of the Academy of Nutrition and Dietetics, 117*(2), 251–264. https://doi.org/10.1016/j.jand.2016.09.021

Medical Guardian. (2016, October 26). *The importance of aerobic exercise for seniors.* Medical Guardian. https://www.medicalguardian.com/medical-alert-blog/fitness/the-importance-of-aerobic-exercise-for-seniors

MedlinePlus. (n.d.). *Exercise clothing and shoes: MedlinePlus Medical Encyclopedia.* Medlineplus.gov. Retrieved February 12, 2022, from https://medlineplus.gov/ency/patientinstructions/000817.htm

MedlinePlus. (2017). *Aging changes in the bones, muscles, and joints: MedlinePlus Medical Encyclopedia.* Medlineplus.gov. https://medlineplus.gov/ency/article/004015.htm

Metkus, T. S. (2014). *Being active when you have heart disease: MedlinePlus Medical Encyclopedia.* Medlineplus.gov. https://medlineplus.gov/ency/patientinstructions/000094.htm

Muscles of the back. (n.d.). TeachMeAnatomy. https://teachmeanatomy.info/back/muscles/

Najafi, L. (2020, November 20). *These dumbbell sets are expert-recommended and in stock*. NBC News. https://www.nbcnews.com/select/shopping/best-dumbbells-home-ncna1184726

National Institutes of Health. (2017). *Vitamin D*. Nih.gov. https://ods.od.nih.gov/factsheets/VitaminD-HealthProfessional/

Pelucchi, C., Bosetti, C., Galeone, C., and La Vecchia, C. (2014). Dietary acrylamide and cancer risk: An updated meta-analysis. *International Journal of Cancer, 136*(12), 2912–2922. https://doi.org/10.1002/ijc.29339

Physiopedia. (2019). *Muscle function: Effects of aging*. Physiopedia. https://www.physio-pedia.com/Muscle_Function:_effects_of_aging

Purposed Physical Therapy. (n.d.). *Keeping my shoulders healthy as I age*. www.purposedphysicaltherapy.com. Retrieved February 22, 2022, from https://www.purposedphysicaltherapy.com/Newsletters/Full-Articles/Keeping-My-Shoulders-Healthy-As-I-Age/a~17546/article.html

Rad, A. (2022, February 15). *Types of movements in the human body*. Kenhub. https://www.kenhub.com/en/library/anatomy/types-of-movements-in-the-human-body

Roland, J. (2020, February 25). *Leg muscles: Thigh and calf muscles, and causes of pain*. Healthline. https://www.healthline.com/health/leg-muscles

Scarpellini, E., Lauritano, E. C., Lupascu, A., Petruzzellis, C., Novi, M. L., Roccarina, D., Gabrielli, M., Serricchio, M., Gasbarrini, G., & Gasbarrini, A. (2007). Efficacy of butyrate in the treatment of diarrhoea-predominant irritable bowel syndrome. *Digestive and Liver Disease Supplements, 1*(1), 19–22. https://doi.org/10.1016/s1594-5804(08)60006-6

Schein, C. (2020, February 28). *The importance of staying hydrated for seniors.* Aegis Living. https://www.aegisliving.com/resource-center/the-importance-of-staying-hydrated/

Scioscia, T. (2017, August 24). *Back muscles and low back pain.* Spine-Health. https://www.spine-health.com/conditions/spine-anatomy/back-muscles-and-low-back-pain

Seguin, R., & Nelson, M. E. (2003). The benefits of strength training for older adults. *American Journal of Preventive Medicine, 25*(3), 141–149. https://doi.org/10.1016/s0749-3797(03)00177-6

Sheff, B. (2016). Your lungs and exercise. *Breathe, 12*(1), 97–100. https://doi.org/10.1183/20734735.elf121

Sissons, C. (2020, May 27). *What percentage of the human body is water?* www.medicalnewstoday.com. https://www.medicalnewstoday.com/articles/what-percentage-of-the-human-body-is-water

TeachMeAnatomy. (2014). *The Intermediate Back Muscles.* Teachmeanatomy.info. https://teachmeanatomy.info/back/muscles/intermediate/

Tripodi, N. (2021, July 6). *What is the posterior chain?* Melbourne Osteopathy Sports Injury Centre. https://www.melbourneosteopathycentre.com.au/blog/training/what-is-the-posterior-chain/

Tucker, A. (2019, January 3). *10 things to do before and after a workout to get better results.* Self. https://www.self.com/story/8-things-to-do-before-and-after-a-workout-to-get-better-results

Vancruze, R. (2018, October 28). *5 best ways to develop a winning mindset.* Vancruzer. https://vancruzer.com/develop-a-winning-mindset/

Waehner, P. (2020, December 23). *Work your chest muscles to burn more calories.* Verywell Fit. https://www.verywellfit.com/your-best-chest-1229817